Of Character

Building Assets in Recovery

Denise D. Crosson, Ph.D.

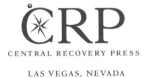

CENTRAL RECOVERY PRESS

LAS VEGAS, NEVADA

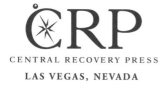

CENTRAL RECOVERY PRESS

LAS VEGAS, NEVADA

CENTRAL RECOVERY PRESS

Central Recovery Press (CRP) is committed to publishing exceptional
material addressing addiction treatment and recovery, including original
and quality books, audio/visual communications, and web-based
new media. Through a diverse selection of titles, it seeks to impact
the behavioral healthcare field with a broad range of unique resources
for professionals, recovering individuals, and their families. For more
information, visit www.centralrecoverypress.com.

CRP donates a portion of its proceeds to *Foundation for Recovery*, a
nonprofit organization local and national in scope. Its purpose is to
promote recovery from addiction through a variety of forums, such as
direct services, research and development, education, study of recovery
alternatives, public awareness, and advocacy.

Central Recovery Press, Las Vegas, 89129
© 2009 by Central Recovery Press, Las Vegas, NV
All rights reserved. Published 2009.
Printed in the United States of America.

16 15 14 13 12 11 10 09   1 2 3 4 5

ISBN 13: 978-0-9799869-2-5 (paperback)
ISBN 10: 0-9799869-2-3

Book design: Sara Streifel, Think Creative Design

For Phillip and Sydney

The two people I miss most
and who taught me the most about character.

For Janet Younger

Who taught me to have fun thinking about how we think,
and who taught me to always take
my clinical opportunities and duties seriously,
but never to take myself too seriously.

CONTENTS

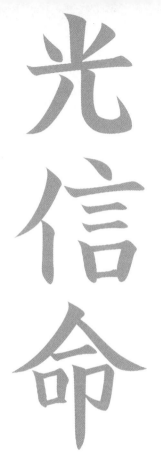

INTRODUCTION

This is a book about character—what it is and what shapes it. *Oxford Dictionary of English* defines character as "the mental and moral qualities distinctive to an individual." Most experts accept this definition, but there is some disagreement on how character is formed. Many argue character is shaped by genetics and experience. While this may be true to some degree, I believe a large part of character can be influenced or created by our choices and our willingness to examine and accept the consequences of those choices.

I believe character is about setting a standard for behavior and then considering whether that standard has been met. When we fail to meet the standard we've set for ourselves, we must examine the situation and our thoughts and feelings to determine why we failed.

For me, self-centered fear exerts enough power to interfere with who I want to be. Acknowledging this allows me to consider what I might learn from the times I did not act as I would have liked. I gain peace and faith by realizing I am guided and protected; and therefore, I have a better chance of facing my fear the next time it arises. When I am able to do that, I am better able to act spiritually rather than allow myself to be controlled by fear.

My interest in character arose years ago as a young nurse. I entered a hospital elevator occupied by a housekeeping worker and a couple with their newborn. The housekeeper was someone I had vaguely noticed for several years. She was a young woman with Down syndrome. What little I knew about her included that she was always at work, had won several awards for perfect attendance, was always pleasant and cheerful, was always willing to help out no matter what the task, and was hard-working and efficient as a housekeeper. I could tell her days off because when she was working, the patients' rooms were cleaner and more orderly.

I had seen her several times calmly talking with patients—sometimes as she worked and other times sitting quietly. I remember wondering if anyone else had caught her doing this, would she get in trouble since housekeeping staff were not expected to talk with patients. I decided it was not my business and didn't say anything about it. I figured she was protected since she cleaned so much better than anyone else and was the most reliable employee on the housekeeping staff.

In the hospital elevator, I watched the housekeeper tell the new parents how beautiful their baby was. The parents smiled nervously and responded with a "thank you." The baby was awake and seemed to be steadily looking at the housekeeper. When she reached out to give the baby her finger, the mother recoiled and withdrew the carrier containing the baby. I watched the hurt and confusion register on the housekeeper's face and saw how embarrassed the father was that I had witnessed the mother's reaction. He started to say something then stammered and stopped.

I made what felt like a superhuman effort to control the anger that suddenly arose within me even though I did not completely understand it. Thankfully what I said was: "Oh, I'm sure you haven't met Jane (name changed to protect anonymity). She is our most dedicated housekeeping worker. She's a good part of the reason why your baby is leaving the hospital healthy and free of infection. Protecting your baby from strangers is a great start at parenting, but Jane isn't really a stranger. She's seen your baby and cleaned her isolette in the nursery every day since she was born. She just wanted to say goodbye and wish you good luck." Both parents visibly relaxed and the mother offered the baby back immediately for a brief contact with the housekeeper. Happily, everyone left the elevator smiling.

The incident was over in minutes, but it highlights the opportunities and pitfalls we are offered in life by character or the lack there of. What exactly were the parents' fears of having a hospital employee touch their infant in the elevator? They had to be aware that numerous other hospital employees—known and unknown to them—had touched their infant while she was hospitalized. Why were they unconcerned about those touches, but concerned about a largely social and friendly encounter they could supervise? Were they afraid because the person was a housekeeper, which might mean her hands were dirty? Were they afraid someone with Down syndrome might impart bad luck? Maybe they feared Down syndrome was contagious? Why were they willing to take my word that it was safe to allow the touch? Why were they willing to accept my character or authority to such an extent that they ignored their prior alarm about the housekeeper's touch? Were they really reassured or did they feel pressured to act as I thought they should?

As I look back, it surprises me that I so clearly recall and retain so much from such a brief encounter. The choices and actions of the people involved in this blink-of-an-eye moment have, over the years, influenced an incredible portion of my character. When I reflect on my anger at the actions of the parents, I am able to see the times I acted just as fearful and biased. To be angry at them was to be angry at myself. While I did not share the same fear of the housekeeper, I had other fears that were just as baseless. My fears and prejudices influenced my behavior in the world just as the parents' had, and those fears had consequences for blameless others as well.

Every time I wanted to recoil in fear from someone or something unknown to me, I have recalled those parents and prayed to act as I had in that elevator incident. I prayed I might reassure myself or seek reassurance from my higher power and not react in baseless fear. Sometimes I have succeeded, other times I have failed. However, over time I have improved and made progress. For me, that improvement is the essence of character.

I believe developing character is using what we have to rise above the limits we impose upon ourselves because of fear, greed, selfishness, and hatred. Character is looking hard for who we are at our most ideal and essential level and doing our best to honor that ideal in everything we do. This book is an attempt to help me continue to do that as I write these reflections. I hope to help you do the same—if you choose.

Accepting

The process or fact of receiving someone or something
as adequate, valid, or suitable.

Denise D. Crosson, Ph.D., RN, FNP-CS

• • •

"HOW FAR YOU GO IN LIFE DEPENDS ON
YOUR BEING TENDER WITH THE YOUNG,
COMPASSIONATE WITH THE AGED,
SYMPATHETIC WITH THE STRIVING,
AND TOLERANT OF THE WEAK AND STRONG.
BECAUSE SOMEDAY IN LIFE
YOU WILL HAVE BEEN ALL OF THESE."

GEORGE WASHINGTON CARVER

When we are accepting in recovery, we "receive" others, the world, our circumstances, and ourselves "as adequate." This does not mean we must be content with things exactly as they are. It means we learn to align ourselves with and acknowledge reality. Only when we have done so are we able to develop the wisdom to know when we can work to change things and when we must learn to accept things as they are.

Too often acceptance is confused with tolerance. Acceptance, in regard to character, is actively reaching out for an understanding that suspends judgment in favor of better knowing another person or ourselves. Tolerance implies a passive and negative attitude or "putting up" with something or someone we are too polite to snub. In asking people whether they would like to be tolerated or accepted, undoubtedly you would find few, if any, who would want to be tolerated. Virtually everyone would want to be accepted.

Accepting others as they are does not mean we must endure unacceptable judgments or actions from them. It means, without anger or retaliation, we acknowledge our powerlessness over the judgments and actions of others. When we make this acknowledgement, we find it easier to accept ourselves even with our imperfections. In turn, when we accept ourselves as whole and adequate, we are more able to enjoy relations with others and accept their humanness and imperfections. Another gift of acceptance is when we are able to accept ourselves, we find the judgment of others often loses its sting.

MEDITATIVE THOUGHT

As I go through life,
help me be more accepting of others,
the world, my circumstances, and myself.
Help me make the extra effort to be accepting,
rather than tolerant, of others.

Adventurous

Willing to take risks or
to try out new methods,
ideas, or experiences.

*Oxford Dictionary of English**

• • •

"IF I HAD TO LIVE MY LIFE AGAIN,
I'D MAKE ALL THE SAME MISTAKES,
ONLY SOONER."

TALLULAH BANKHEAD

Being adventurous means being willing to try new things. What often hampers our adventurousness is fear of being wrong or making mistakes. It's true that following our inclinations sometimes means we will make mistakes; but making mistakes isn't always bad. Often we learn more and better remember how to do something correctly from the experience of having done it incorrectly once.

Being adventurous allows us to try things other people enjoy, to see if we like those things, too. It allows us to see or hear of an activity or idea and explore it to determine if it adds to our lives. An adventurous spirit means being open to the present moment and stepping out in faith. Does this mean we let anyone who offers teach us how to skydive? Probably not. Being adventurous does not mean ignoring risks inherent in an activity or idea. It means considering the possible benefits of trying something new in healthy balance with consideration of the risks involved.

MEDITATIVE THOUGHT

HELP ME ENJOY AND EXERCISE MY ADVENTUROUS SPIRIT
IN A BALANCED AND HEALTHY WAY.
RELIEVE ME OF THE SELF-CENTERED FEAR
THAT HAMPERS MY JOY IN LIFE.

Affectionate

Readily feeling or showing
fondness or tenderness.
*Oxford Dictionary of English**

• • •

"BEGINNING TODAY, TREAT EVERYONE YOU MEET,
FRIEND OR FOE, LOVED ONE OR STRANGER,
AS IF THEY WERE GOING TO BE DEAD AT MIDNIGHT.
EXTEND TO EACH PERSON,
NO MATTER HOW TRIVIAL THE CONTACT,
ALL THE CARE AND KINDNESS AND UNDERSTANDING
AND LOVE THAT YOU CAN MUSTER,
AND DO IT WITH NO THOUGHT OF ANY REWARD.
YOUR LIFE WILL NEVER BE THE SAME AGAIN."

OG MANDINO**

Another definition of affection is the expression of unconditional positive regard for another. Most often we show affection to people we know and love, but affection can be shown toward people we encounter in our daily lives whether we have ongoing relationships with them or not.

Expressing affection can be as simple as listening to a friend; giving someone a warm, sincere hug; offering a moment of real presence and a smile to someone we don't know, but whom we sense may need it; or even buying a book or cookies we know a friend would enjoy for no reason other than we thought of her at that moment.

Affection is a way of showing we are grateful for the gifts in our lives that are our friends and family. Affection is not a contract. It is not expressed with the thought of what we will get in return. Sometimes, only we will know if we are expressing genuine affection or if our actions are intended to control or manipulate. We will know, however, if and when "giving" feels wrong to us in recovery. We can pay attention to our motives in all our actions in our relationships as we do our daily Tenth Step.

We also should be attentive to the costs of selfishly motivated giving. The costs usually include feeling isolated and alone, unknown by others, disappointed and resentful when our expectations are not met, or strangely hollow when we get what we think we wanted. In contrast, sincere affection connects us to the person we love specifically, and, often, to humanity in general. Affection makes us feel content, fulfilled, and liked by others for who we are rather than for what we do.

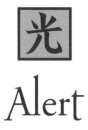

Alert

Quick to notice any unusual and potentially
dangerous or difficult circumstances; vigilant.

Oxford Dictionary of English*

• • •

"NO METHOD NOR DISCIPLINE CAN SUPERSEDE
THE NECESSITY OF BEING FOREVER ON THE ALERT.
WHAT IS A COURSE OF HISTORY, OR PHILOSOPHY,
OR POETRY, NO MATTER HOW WELL SELECTED,
OR THE BEST SOCIETY, OR THE MOST
ADMIRABLE ROUTINE OF LIFE, COMPARED WITH
THE DISCIPLINE OF LOOKING ALWAYS AT WHAT IS TO BE SEEN?
WILL YOU BE A READER, A STUDENT MERELY, OR A SEER?
READ YOUR FATE, SEE WHAT IS BEFORE YOU,
AND WALK ON INTO FUTURITY."

HENRY DAVID THOREAU

At first it may appear alertness has little to do with character. However, many other aspects of character tend to mean little when we are not alert.

If we are kind, but not alert to opportunities to demonstrate kindness to those we love, we often end up being kinder to a stranger than to our spouse or children. If we are not alert and responsive to our feelings and life circumstances, we are less able to be present and honest with ourselves about our motives, choices, and behavior.

Like all character assets, being alert in its extreme—hyper-vigilance—can cause as many problems as it solves. In hyper-vigilance we are more likely to overreact to people and circumstances, acting in situations where no action is required. In recovery, we strive for balance, seeking to be calmly and respectfully alert to people and the world around us without hyper-vigilance or fear.

MEDITATIVE THOUGHT

HELP ME BE CALMLY PRESENT
AND ALERT AS I LIVE MY LIFE.

Altruism

Disinterested and selfless concern
for the well-being of others.

Oxford Dictionary of English*

• • •

"MY DEFINITION OF ALTRUISM IS:
BE WISELY SELFISH AND KNOW THAT YOUR HAPPINESS
DEPENDS ON THE HAPPINESS OF THOSE AROUND YOU
AND THE WORLD IN GENERAL. IF SOCIETY SUFFERS
YOU WILL SUFFER, SO LOVE YOURSELF ENOUGH
TO WORK FOR THE SOCIAL GOOD."

DALAI LAMA**

Altruism is when we do something helpful or generous for someone without expecting anything in return. When we are altruistic, we are not interested in controlling situations, getting credit for our actions, avoiding blame, atoning for wrongs, or appearing to be someone we are not. When we are altruistic, we want to contribute from the generous gifts so freely given to us in recovery, to the world in general, or someone in particular.

When we are altruistic, our hearts are open to the needs of the world and others, as well as daily opportunities to make our part of the world better. Whether anyone notices, our lives are made better by an altruistic attitude. It is not possible to live altruistically without being powerfully affected by the appreciation of our connection to the world and others.

When we are altruistic, we allow a loving higher power to use us as a channel for the light and love that saved us from active addiction. In doing that, we give back to the world we harmed in active addiction, and our humanity is restored. We are a living amend.

MEDITATIVE THOUGHT

HELP ME GO THROUGH MY DAY WITH GREATER AWARENESS
OF OPPORTUNITIES FOR ALTRUISTIC ACTION.
HELP ME BE GRATEFULLY AWARE OF THE RESTORATION
OF MY HUMANITY IN RECOVERY.

Ambitious

(Of a plan or a piece of work)
intended to satisfy high aspirations
and therefore difficult to achieve.

Oxford Dictionary of English*

• • •

"WITHOUT AMBITION ONE STARTS NOTHING.
WITHOUT WORK ONE FINISHES NOTHING.
THE PRIZE WILL NOT BE SENT TO YOU.
YOU HAVE TO WIN IT."

RALPH WALDO EMERSON

Ambition is the combination of effort, commitment, and willingness to risk failure in order to accomplish more. Being ambitious means extending ourselves to grow, learn, or do more. As in all character assets, balance in ambition is important. Too much ambition may drive us to try too hard, to exert ourselves to no good purpose, or twist our characters to succeed at any price. Too little ambition may lead to stagnation and complacency. Neither of these extremes is comfortable or likely to enhance our recovery.

In contrast, a healthy degree of ambition, mixed with the willingness to laugh at ourselves and learn, will enrich our lives and the lives of others by helping us make each day our own. Without ambition we may succeed more often, but we may stretch less and enjoy life less. Being ambitious means we may fail more often, making other character assets such as balance, patience, and gentleness with ourselves even more important. We need to keep in mind that we may fail more often because we are making more effort and commitment.

MEDITATIVE THOUGHT

HELP ME BE AMBITIOUS IN RECOVERY AND LIFE,
WITH BALANCE, PATIENCE, AND A SENSE OF HUMOR.

Attentive

Paying close attention to something;
assiduously attending to the comfort
or wishes of others;
very polite or courteous.
Oxford Dictionary of English*

• • •

"A GOOD LISTENER IS NOT ONLY POPULAR EVERYWHERE,
BUT AFTER A WHILE HE GETS TO KNOW SOMETHING."
WILSON MIZNER**

Being attentive is more than listening, but it is impossible to be attentive without listening. In recovery, we learn to attend to others by attending to ourselves. We spent years using drugs to quiet the inner wisdom that questioned what we were doing to ourselves and those we loved. We used drugs and demanded that others take care of us or pay the price of our addiction with us or for us.

In recovery, we learn that to honestly give anything to another we must have it ourselves. We cannot love another without self-love. When we try to take a shortcut to love and to feeling better by loving someone without self-love, we trade affection or approval for honest connection. This is more like a business transaction than a relationship; one where we say "I'll give you love if you don't mention…" or "I'll be your lover if you spend all your time with me to distract me from the work I need to do or the pain I feel."

Attending is the same. We cannot honestly be attentive to another person without learning to attend to ourselves. When we're not attentive we are listening with only half an ear; never really thinking of or feeling the impact of what another is sharing with us. When we do this, we rob ourselves of the full benefit of the therapeutic value of one addict helping another.

Calm

Not showing or feeling nervousness, anger,
or other strong emotions; make (someone)
tranquil and quiet; soothe.

*Oxford Dictionary of English**

• • •

"CALM SOUL OF ALL THINGS! MAKE IT MINE
TO FEEL, AMID THE CITY'S JAR,
THAT THERE ABIDES A PEACE OF THINE,
MAN DID NOT MAKE, AND CANNOT MAR!"

MATTHEW ARNOLD

Feeling calm is easy in the right setting. In active addiction, we sought to make anywhere the right setting by using drugs to change how we felt or change our perceptions of where we were. In recovery, we seek to be calm.

Real calm cannot be created or destroyed by external circumstances or other people's reactions. Calm is a character asset developed through disciplined practice and experience working the Twelve Steps, praying, and meditating. It is the ability to know we are okay even when we feel hopeless or sad. It is the gift that empowers us to do the right thing even when we don't feel like it or when we think doing anything is a waste of time.

Being calm gives us the ability to sit with our feelings, whether those

By permission of Oxford University Press. © 1998, 1999, 2001, 2003 by Oxford University Press.

feelings are joyous or painful and know we are more than what we feel at that moment. Being calm helps us remember we are guided and protected. It helps us know that despite whatever is happening, no matter how painful, we will find the strength to continue. It lets us talk with others about the pain we have or the joy we experience. In doing this, our ability to be calm grows as we become more connected with the world and people in our lives.

Curiously, in recovery, we grow more engaged with the people and things we love and more detached from them at the same time. In calm, we are able to appreciate this moment of our life more fully and let it go with grace.

MEDITATIVE THOUGHT

Help me be calm even when
I feel troubled or excited.
As I live my life, help me engage
more fully in the present moment
and then let it go.

Candid

Truthful and straightforward; frank.
Oxford Dictionary of English*

• • •

"BY CANDOR WE ARE NOT TO UNDERSTAND TRIFLING
AND UNCALLED FOR EXPOSITIONS OF TRUTH;
BUT A SENTIMENT THAT PROVES A CONVICTION
OF THE NECESSITY OF SPEAKING TRUTH,
WHEN SPEAKING AT ALL...."

JAMES FENIMORE COOPER

When we are candid, we provide relevant information in a situation or relationship. Being candid often can encourage spontaneous honest disclosure. Sometimes, in recovery, this is the self-disclosure that saves our lives. Other times, being candid means saying something that is hard for us to say; perhaps it is the honest disclosure of seeing something in others that concerns us.

Though often difficult, being candid has advantages. When we are candid, there are no secrets that own us or take away from our peace in recovery. If we are candid, we are well and well known by the people in our lives. This means the connections we have are deep, rich, and able to sustain us and our loved ones. It means the people who love us can help us in difficult times and celebrate with us in joyous times because they know and understand us on a more intimate level.

Being candid is one of the greatest protections we have in recovery. It helps us fight relapse. It means we are in regular contact with people who know us and will tell us when they see evidence of active addiction in our thinking or behavior.

Caring

Displaying kindness and concern for others;
the work or practice of looking after those
unable to care for themselves,
especially the sick and the elderly.

*Oxford Dictionary of English**

• • •

"LOVE SEEKETH NOT ITSELF TO PLEASE,
NOR FOR ITSELF HATH ANY CARE,
BUT FOR ANOTHER GIVES ITS EASE,
AND BUILDS A HEAVEN IN HELL'S DESPAIR."

WILLIAM BLAKE

Many mistakenly limit caring to doing for someone only what he or she wants done. Caring also can involve doing for or with someone, something he or she may *not* want done, but desperately needs.

One of the better definitions of caring can be found in a book for nurse managers. It says the essence of nursing is to help a patient, whether ill or well, live as independently as possible by helping him perform the daily activities he would otherwise perform if he had the necessary strength and ability. This concept is a very workable definition in recovery since we are confronted with a chronic, incurable, and fatal illness that tells us we do not have a disease. Those who care about others, as well as themselves, will offer assistance in such a way that usually will provide a recovery-oriented solution.

At times, caring means telling someone we love something that will make him or her angry, but may provide that person with some combination of the strength, will, and knowledge needed to stay clean. Other times caring may mean spending a relaxing afternoon with a friend. Knowing what is required in a situation comes with the experience and willingness to work a recovery program that gives us perspective and wisdom.

24

Character

The mental and moral qualities
distinctive to an individual.
Oxford Dictionary of English*

• • •

"IT IS NOT IN THE STILL CALM OF LIFE,
OR THE REPOSE OF A PACIFIC STATION,
THAT GREAT CHARACTERS ARE FORMED....
GREAT NECESSITIES CALL OUT GREAT VIRTUES."

ABIGAIL ADAMS

What is character? Character is doing the right thing for the right reason even when it's hard or unpopular. Character is doing what you think is best even when others will not understand. Character is acknowledging when you are wrong and learning the lessons from that acknowledgement. Character frees you from the need to be right or popular. Character is about what you do when you know no one is watching or how you conduct yourself when you know someone trusts you enough not to check up on you. Character is what helps you sleep well even when things are not going perfectly. Character is the combination of personality and behavior that when well and consistently practiced makes for a life worth living. Character is the most important, and sometimes least noticed, contribution

By permission of Oxford University Press. © 1998, 1999, 2001, 2003 by Oxford University Press.

you make to your family and friends, community, the world, and yourself.

No one can take away good character; only you can give, sell, or throw it away. Character is what you have left when others look at your life and think you have lost everything. Character is what lets you enjoy being at the top of the world or an "overnight success" without losing perspective because you know that external success is not everything. Character is what prevents you from behaving in oppressive or one-down thinking about others when you are successful. Character is what stops you from thinking of yourself as one-down when you are presently not successful by external standards.

MEDITATIVE THOUGHT

As I live my life, help me take stock of my character.
Help me appreciate and gratefully enjoy my assets.
Help me be willing to become more aware
and ask for removal of my defects,
then give me the strength to act on my assets.

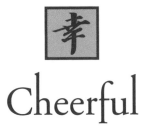

Cheerful

Noticeably happy and optimistic.
Oxford Dictionary of English*

• • •

"...SAY LITTLE AND DO MUCH;
AND RECEIVE ALL MEN
WITH A CHEERFUL COUNTENANCE."

SHAMMAI, TALMUD, MISHNAH, *PIRQEI AVOT 1:15*

Cheerfulness of character is easily recognized by the peace and joy those who have it take in daily life. Sometimes being cheerful simply means noticing and expressing how well one's day is going. Other times it means deciding that since something must be done or is the right thing to do, doing it cheerfully is the best and easiest way to go about it. We all have times when what needs to be done is not what we really want to do.

Cheerfulness in doing that "necessary thing" is what separates people with character.

People without the cheer of character let external circumstances decide how they will feel and act, and what their attitude will be, rather than deciding they are independent of external events. This is not to suggest external events don't have an effect on us in recovery. It means we recognize and claim the freedom and responsibility to choose our attitude, response, and behavior from a perspective that includes appreciation of who we are.

This does not imply we act happy when we are sad or troubled, for this would not be honest. Instead, we acknowledge and ask for support to help us accept our feelings. Being cheerful means we move on without the grumbling and complaining many of us practiced when we grudgingly did something we resented.

Doing the right thing resentfully does not qualify as doing the right thing for the right reason. Resentment robs us of the benefits of doing the right thing. It takes away any peace that might be possible for us and those around us.

HELP ME ACKNOWLEDGE AND DEAL WITH MY LIFE CIRCUMSTANCES
WITH A REALISTIC APPRECIATION OF WHO I AM
SEPARATE FROM THOSE CIRCUMSTANCES.
HELP ME DO THE RIGHT THING FOR THE RIGHT REASON
WITHOUT RESENTMENT AND WITH THE CHEER OF CHARACTER.

Committed

(Be committed to) to be dedicated to something;
pledge or set aside (resources) for future use;
be in a long-term emotional relationship with (someone).

*Oxford Dictionary of English**

• • •

"COMING TOGETHER IS A BEGINNING,
STAYING TOGETHER IS PROGRESS,
AND WORKING TOGETHER IS SUCCESS."

HENRY FORD

In active addiction, many of us could only be committed to getting and using drugs. If we felt commitment to other people, ideas, or institutions, acting on the commitment was often impossible because of the demands of our disease. This lack of commitment to others and ourselves often translated into having a life devoid of meaning. Without the foundation commitment provides, our lives often drifted on the currents of our disease.

In recovery, we first learn about commitment through our commitment to recovery. As we grow and work the Twelve Steps, we develop meaningful commitments to ourselves, others, and the world. From these commitments flow the opportunity to live a life that has meaning; a life with a foundation we develop from writing a searching and fearless moral inventory. In the process of that inventory we get to decide what our values and commitments are, as well as the general direction and purpose we want for our lives.

Being committed to someone else, something else, or ourselves requires much of us. It requires we accept uncertainty in our lives, as well as the uncertainty of who our friend or lover will become as he or she grows and changes in ways unknown to us. It requires we give of ourselves to support an idea or institution we believe is important. Often this is required even when the idea is not popular or the institution seems unlikely to succeed.

Being committed requires the consistency and fortitude to do what is required even when we are tired or don't feel we can. The rewards of commitment include more connections with other people, more certainty about the purpose of our lives and our ideals and beliefs, acceptance of the uncertainty of living in the here and now, more peace and happiness, an enhanced ability to withstand adversity, and quiet self-confidence.

The essential question when it comes to commitment is: Are we better or worse for having nothing in our lives that is important enough for us to stand up for?

Compassionate

Showing empathetic concern for the sufferings
or misfortunes of others.

Denise D. Crosson, Ph.D., RN, FNP-CS

• • •

"I HAVE STRIVEN NOT TO LAUGH AT HUMAN ACTIONS,
NOT TO WEEP AT THEM, NOR TO HATE THEM,
BUT TO UNDERSTAND THEM."

BARUCH SPINOZA

Compassion is easier to see when it occurs than to describe when it does not. Too often we think of being compassionate as being nice to everyone, especially those who are less fortunate than us. That attitude is more like condescension and smugness than true compassion. Compassion is not about being or trying to "make nice." It is the attentive, respectful acknowledgement of the basic humanness of all people, particularly those who anger, frighten, or harm us.

When our attention is focused on someone we like, trust, or love, our behavior is more consistent with kindness, love, or friendship than compassion. It is usually easy to behave compassionately with a friend or lover who is in pain. The compassion of character is the compassion we show those we don't know or who offend us. This compassion is the behavioral acknowledgment that all beings want the same thing—happiness and freedom from suffering. It is the behavioral commitment to not make things worse for someone who is suffering even when we don't like or trust him or her. At best, it is the ability to behave in a helpful manner in such a situation.

Compassion is one of the most powerful ways we have of improving our world. When we behave compassionately to those expecting anger or retaliation, we disturb their view of the world and of us in a way that may promote growth and encourage human connection.

MEDITATIVE THOUGHT

HELP ME ACT COMPASSIONATELY
EVEN WHEN I AM DISTURBED BY ANOTHER.

Considerate

Careful not to inconvenience or harm others.

Oxford Dictionary of English*

• • •

"During my second month of nursing school, our professor gave us a pop quiz. I was a conscientious student and had breezed through the questions, until I read the last one:

'What is the first name of the woman who cleans the school?'

Surely this was some kind a joke. I had seen the cleaning woman several times. She was tall, dark-haired, and in her 50s, but how would I know her name? I handed in my paper, leaving the last question blank. Before class ended, one student asked if the last question would count toward our quiz grade. "Absolutely," said the professor.

"In your careers, you will meet many people.
All are significant.
They deserve your attention and care,
even if all you do is smile and say 'Hello'."
I've never forgotten that lesson.
I also learned her name was Dorothy."

Joann C. Jones

Consideration for others was not a strong suit for most of us during active addiction. We usually were guided by whatever helped us get and use drugs. In recovery, we learn, usually by having it shown to us, the meaning of consideration. Being considerate may mean holding a door open for someone whose hands are full. It may mean letting someone out of a tricky traffic situation without animosity.

Other times consideration requires more of us. It may mean putting our desires aside to support another addict or someone we love. The easy, natural, and anonymous consideration we show in traffic situations or in holding a door open for someone is the easiest to master.

The more difficult consideration—the kind that costs us something we want—is harder. This is because showing consideration in these instances makes us vulnerable.

While consideration makes our commitment and love visible to those important to us, being considerate in other situations may make us feel defenseless. In those cases we must have a real internalization and comfort with our own powerlessness.

When we practice consideration that makes us vulnerable we strengthen our First Step acknowledgement of our powerlessness, and in doing so we claim our strength. The strength that says we are secure enough in our recovery to risk being vulnerable and risk being hurt.

HELP ME NOTICE AND RESPOND TO THE OPPORTUNITIES TO BE CONSIDERATE THAT ARE PRESENTED TO ME TODAY.
HELP ME UTILIZE WHATEVER DISCOMFORT I FEEL IN BEING VULNERABLE TO STRENGTHEN AND INTERNALIZE MY ADMISSION OF POWERLESSNESS.

Cooperative

Involving mutual assistance in working towards
a common goal; willing to be of assistance.

Oxford Dictionary of English *

• • •

"GREAT DISCOVERIES AND IMPROVEMENTS INVARIABLY
INVOLVE THE COOPERATION OF MANY MINDS.
I MAY BE GIVEN CREDIT FOR HAVING BLAZED THE TRAIL,
BUT WHEN I LOOK AT THE SUBSEQUENT DEVELOPMENTS
I FEEL THE CREDIT IS DUE TO OTHERS RATHER THAN TO MYSELF."

ALEXANDER GRAHAM BELL

In active addiction, we seldom worked in cooperation with anyone on anything other than ways to get or use drugs. Even if we were able to cooperate with others in some settings, our motivation and abilities were almost certainly adversely affected by our disease.

One of the most important ways we learn about cooperation in recovery is in service to others. Too often cooperation gets confused with submission, which subverts true cooperation, for it is not possible to work toward the same end without having agreement about what is being sought.

One of the simplest ways we learn to cooperate is in carrying a message to other addicts who suffer. This is made simple for us by our respect for the traditions of our recovery fellowship. In service, because we start from the assumption of our primary purpose, the only consensus we need to reach is the best means of accomplishing our goal of carrying a message of recovery.

This does not mean cooperation is effortless or easy, though it helps us with structure. By learning to cooperate in service, we may gradually become better at cooperation in circumstances where the goal of our actions must be decided in consultation with others. When we do this, we are less likely to end up dug in and defending a position that places us in conflict.

The benefits of cooperation include a greater sense of connection with others, greater productivity, and a quiet sense of pride. Cooperation serves to make our lives richer by ensuring we never need to feel alone. Cooperating can often make certain projects or tasks easier, fun, and possible. Cooperation extends our sphere of influence without feeding our unhealthy desire for control.

Courageous

Not deterred by danger or pain; brave.
*Oxford Dictionary of English**

• • •

"WHAT WOULD LIFE BE
IF WE HAD NO COURAGE TO ATTEMPT ANYTHING?"
VINCENT VAN GOGH

Most of us never drew a courageous breath while in active addiction. We often spent our time absorbed in fear about things that never happened. We may have acted brave in an attempt to fool ourselves and others into thinking we were courageous. Under that bravado, however, we usually were fearful and knew our actions were hollow.

In recovery, we begin to know courage by watching and respecting others who tell us they are afraid and then find the spiritual and emotional resources to walk through their fear to do the right thing. With their help we learn to do this as well.

Courage of character demands we consciously consider all things that are frightening to us over which we have no control—the disease of addiction, death, loss of important relationships, unjust treatment by others and institutions, accidents, weather, and other disasters.

Courage of character requires we acknowledge our fears, and then surrender them to our higher power so we may act courageously in matters over which we do have power. If we never acknowledge the fears outside our control, we use too much energy trying to distract ourselves from the possibility of impending doom.

When we acknowledge and face these fears, energy is freed for other spiritual pursuits.

Courage of character is sometimes evident when we stand alone and represent an unpopular position. More commonly it is evident in the courage it takes to face ourselves, our disease, and our daily lives. The courage to stand for something, even when alone, comes from the use of courage in the smaller areas of our lives. It is the daily practice of courage that requires us to be honest with those we love about our less loveable aspects, our mistakes, and our fears. In doing this, we learn enough about our assets and limitations to sustain us in situations requiring a more dramatic display of courage. Sometimes this means telling our employer we can't do something because it conflicts with a moral duty we owe elsewhere. Sometimes this means honestly self-reporting a serious error to facilitate amending a situation before it worsens.

Few of us will have our courage tested by being on a battlefield out-manned and out-gunned. Yet we all face situations where acting courageously may make the world better and may also place us at some risk. If we tell our employer we cannot do as we've been asked, or report a mistake we've made, we could be fired or disciplined. Doing the right thing even when afraid of consequences is courage.

The gifts of courage are many. Courage lets us look back at our day with appreciation and peace. It frees us from constant fear, worry, and self-doubt. It offers us the opportunity to be humbly satisfied with ourselves.

MEDITATIVE THOUGHT

IN ACTIVE ADDICTION I PRACTICED RECKLESS DISREGARD FOR MYSELF AND OTHERS. IN RECOVERY, HELP ME BE AWARE OF AND GRATEFUL FOR THE OPPORTUNITIES TO PRACTICE COURAGE. AS I EVALUATE MY DAY AND MY ACTIONS, HELP ME BE GRATEFUL FOR THE BENEFITS THAT FLOW FROM MY COURAGE IN LIFE.

Creative

Relating to or involving the use of the imagination
or original ideas to create something.

*Oxford Dictionary of English**

• • •

"IF YOU HAVE BUILT CASTLES IN THE AIR,
YOUR WORK NEED NOT BE LOST;
THAT IS WHERE THEY SHOULD BE.
NOW PUT THE FOUNDATIONS UNDER THEM."

HENRY DAVID THOREAU

Most of us in active addiction were quite imaginative. This often resulted in destructive consequences. We may have come up with ways to separate others from their money or resources so we could get and use more drugs. We may have concocted elaborate lies to justify or explain our actions. Whatever we did with our imagination, we usually ended up loaded, afraid, and alone, often having destroyed something of value. Creativity requires imagination and the creation of something. This second requirement was lacking in active addiction.

In recovery, our imagination, without commitment to creation, can continue to get us into trouble. Even now, with clearer heads, we may use our imagination to avoid work we owe our employer. Most of the time, it is actually easier to just do our job. We may use our imagination to concoct complex reasons why the ordinary rules of good equitable relationships do not apply to us. In practice, this may be diverting and entertaining, but it usually results in damage to others and/or ourselves.

We only can create by working a program of recovery that supports us in avoiding the destruction that is such a common characteristic of our disease.

Creativity in recovery allows us to make connections with others by being able to imagine how they see the world. It allows us to see a number of possible solutions to a problem then select the one that creates the best possible outcome. Creativity in recovery lets us imagine a new career, then work to attain the needed skills to do it. Our progress with creativity must always be inventoried by its consequences. Trying something new and original that does not meet our goals does not count as a creative failure as long as it does not destroy something important. It may actually give us information about how to approach our next creative effort. In contrast, doing something new and original that does meet our goal, but destroys or costs something dear to us would count as a creative failure.

Decisive

Settling an issue; producing a definite result;
having or showing the ability to make decisions
quickly and effectively.

Oxford Dictionary of English*

• • •

"I SAY THAT THE STRONGEST PRINCIPLE OF GROWTH
LIES IN HUMAN CHOICE."

GEORGE ELIOT

Being decisive can be a tricky area for recovering addicts. We were impulsive and dove headlong into situations that were not in our best interest while in active addiction. Too often we come into recovery without a clear idea of the difference between doing something quickly and making a good decision quickly. In order to be decisive in recovery, we must have a clear idea of our values and goals.

We develop clarity about our values by writing an inventory and sharing it with our sponsor. By doing this, we start to understand how the disease of addiction affects our thinking and behavior. We see patterns of how we compromised our values while in the grip of our disease. If we do the work ahead of time—writing the steps and sharing them with a sponsor; examining our thoughts, feelings, motives, and actions on a daily basis; and realizing what works for us in recovery and what we can no longer comfortably do—then being decisive is possible. If we have not done the work required to clean up the wreckage of our active addiction and truly live in recovery, then we are not able to make good decisions consistently and/or quickly.

Even as experienced members with clean time and recovery, it usually is best to check decisions with someone we trust who has our best interests in mind and who will tell us the truth, before moving forward with our decisions. In doing this, we celebrate and practice our recovery. By asking for help, we remind ourselves that we are never alone. We remind ourselves of the importance of being humble enough to seek and consider the counsel of another. We show that we are open-minded and willing to grow.

MEDITATIVE THOUGHT

HELP ME GROW IN MY DECISIVENESS
AS I GROW IN MY RECOVERY.

Determined

Having made a firm decision
and being resolved not to change it.

Oxford Dictionary of English*

• • •

"THERE IS NO CHANCE, NO DESTINY, NO FATE,
CAN CIRCUMVENT, OR HINDER, OR CONTROL
THE FIRM RESOLVE OF A DETERMINED SOUL..."

ELLA WHEELER WILCOX

While determination can be a problem for addicts, it also holds the potential to make our lives fuller and more successful. Determination is different from being stubborn, something that most addicts are naturally. Determination implies firm resolve in a well thought out, worthy course of action. Being stubborn is resolve without regard for facts or context. Determination requires we are clear about what we are doing, why we are doing it, and what the possible outcomes may be. We can, with the help of our sponsor and recovering friends, be fairly certain about our behavior and motives if we use the help available to us.

In recovery, determination can be what gets us to do something difficult, but important, when we feel beaten. It can be what helps us "not give up five minutes before the miracle." This is the determination of character, and we can see how different it is than being stubborn.

Determination requires that at every point along the way, from making our first decision to accomplishing our goal, we remain open to guidance from others and our higher power. Being determined, instead of stubborn, is not easy, but it is possible in recovery and is worth the effort.

Devoted

Very loving or loyal.
*Oxford Dictionary of English**

• • •

"WHERESOEVER YOU GO,
GO WITH ALL YOUR HEART."

CONFUCIUS

Devotion is often thought of as old-fashioned. Nothing, however, could be more necessary in modern life where people move at breakneck speed and objects become obsolete before they are even paid for.

Devotion of character or devotion in the face of uncertainty is the devotion we show when we love another person unconditionally. This is the devotion of the secure and spiritually-grounded person who can be generous, gracious, and loving in the absence of a reward. The benefits of offering love and devotion is not in what one gets back, but in what one gives.

Devotion does not mean accepting abuse. Sometimes this means having the strength and courage to remove ourselves from a harmful or abusive relationship or having the ability to separate the person from his or her unacceptable behavior.

Saying and showing that we love someone while refusing to accept his or her behavior is one of the greatest acts of love one person can perform for another. It shows we have the eyes of devotion that allow us to look past what someone is doing to see who he or she is.

HELP ME DEVELOP MY CAPACITY FOR DEVOTION
EVEN IN THE ABSENCE OF ITS RETURN.

Discernment

The ability to judge well.

*Oxford Dictionary of English**

• • •

"THE FIRST METHOD FOR ESTIMATING
THE INTELLIGENCE OF A RULER
IS TO LOOK AT THE MEN HE HAS AROUND HIM."

NICCOLÒ MACHIAVELLI

Discernment is a character trait common to many, but used by few. In our active addiction, we often had access to the quiet inner voice that said, "Don't do it," or "Maybe I should wait on this." However, we ignored or drugged that inner wisdom into silence. Even in recovery we have so many competing demands on our attention and so many available distractions that ignoring our inner voice is common.

Often we ignore our quiet inner voice because it tells us something we do not want to hear. Then we feel uncertain or unhappy, and we distract ourselves with food, shopping, or gambling.

We distance ourselves from a reality we find too threatening. If we practice being discerning, we listen to our inner guidance and consult with a friend or our sponsor so we can make choices that change the quality of our lives for the better. We can choose to work to improve a damaged relationship or get out of a relationship that is unhealthy or beyond repair. We can delay getting into a business deal that sounds too good to be true until we have checked it out more carefully. In being quietly attentive to our inner wisdom, or discernment, we can avoid paying the consequences of denial, delusion, and distraction.

Empower

Make (someone) stronger and more confident,
especially in controlling their life
and claiming their rights.

Oxford Dictionary of English*

• • •

"THE GREATEST GOOD YOU CAN DO FOR ANOTHER
IS NOT JUST TO SHARE YOUR RICHES,
BUT TO REVEAL TO HIM HIS OWN."

BENJAMIN DISRAELI

In early recovery, sometimes the best we can do regarding empowerment is not to oppress someone else. As we grow in recovery and as our self-awareness and self-assurance increases, we look for ways to empower the people we encounter in our lives.

This may be done by encouraging a loved one to try a new career or return to school and then doing the hard work to help them be successful. It may be an opportunity at work to teach, nurture, and trust a colleague with a project he or she has never done before, and then allow the person to do it and offer help if and when needed.

The opportunity to empower often arises with sponsees and recovering friends when we have experience they lack. When we seek to empower, we help only when asked and where needed.

When we are empowered, we do not need or take credit for work done. If we are thanked for our efforts, we quietly acknowledge how good it feels to facilitate the growth and development of someone we love, making it clear the credit belongs to him or her. We may even express gratitude for the people in our lives who empowered us and taught us to be empowering. By doing this we serve as living examples of the many gifts recovery has to offer.

MEDITATIVE THOUGHT

HELP ME NOTICE AND BE GRATEFUL
FOR THE PEOPLE WHO EMPOWER ME.
HELP ME MAKE THE BEST USE OF MY TALENTS AND ABILITIES
TO EMPOWER THE PEOPLE IN MY LIFE
WHO WANT MY HELP.

Enthusiastic

Having or showing
intense and eager enjoyment,
interest, or approval.
*Oxford Dictionary of English**

• • •

"NOTHING GREAT WAS EVER ACHIEVED
WITHOUT ENTHUSIASM."

RALPH WALDO EMERSON

Enthusiasm is an often contagious joy and energy. Think back to the last time you were with someone who was enthusiastically doing or discussing something. Didn't you pay closer attention to what was being said or done? This is often true even when the activity or topic is not something we are normally interested in or agree with.

It is easier to be enthusiastic when things are going our way. Enthusiasm for life is the emotion that helps us assess our character. Are we able to enthusiastically do hard or painful work to support ourselves and others in recovery even when things are not going our way?

If we are grateful for the opportunity to recover and live based on spiritual principles, then we know that everything, even pain, offers a gift or gifts. We can, at a minimum, be grateful and enthusiastic for the opportunity to be clean and look for the gifts as we do the work necessary to maintain our spiritual condition. When we do our part, our lives in recovery can be filled on a daily basis with this joy and energy.

Forgiving

Allowing room for error or weakness.

Merriam-Webster's Collegiate Dictionary*

• • •

"FORGIVENESS IS BETTER THAN PUNISHMENT;
FOR THE ONE IS THE PROOF OF A GENTLE,
THE OTHER OF A SAVAGE NATURE."

EPICTETUS

Often in active addiction or even before we began using drugs, we hoarded and jealously guarded our resentments. We used them as excuses for our poor choices or shortcomings. "If he hadn't done _____ to me, I would not have _____." Most of us can fill in the blanks without much thought. Being forgiving in recovery requires more effort and honesty than simply looking for a scapegoat. As a result, resentments, the unwillingness to forgive, and the consequences of both often plague us in recovery.

Forgiving helps us far more than it helps the offending party. Once we forgive a wrong done to us, we are free from the pain of resentment, and our lives are no longer controlled by what was done to us. With our mind clear and unclouded by pain and resentment, we are free to learn all the lessons available and move on.

When we forgive another, we acknowledge his or her human fallibility and accept our own. Even

*By permission. From Merriam-Webster's Collegiate® Dictionary, 11th Edition
© 2008 by Merriam-Webster, Incorporated (www.Merriam-Webster.com).*

after we have forgiven others, they still must live with the reality of the harm they caused. As our ability to forgive expands, we find we are able to forgive others much sooner than they are able to forgive themselves. When we can empathize with their pain, our compassion and understanding grows.

Free

Not or no longer confined or imprisoned;
(free of/from) not subject to or affected by (something undesirable);
using or expending something without restraint.

Oxford Dictionary of English*

• • •

"FREEDOM IS NOT MERELY THE CHANCE TO DO AS ONE PLEASES;
NEITHER IS IT MERELY THE OPPORTUNITY
TO CHOOSE BETWEEN SET ALTERNATIVES.
FREEDOM IS, FIRST OF ALL,
THE CHANCE TO FORMULATE THE AVAILABLE CHOICES,
TO ARGUE OVER THEM—
AND THEN, THE OPPORTUNITY TO CHOOSE."

C. WRIGHT MILLS**

The freedom from the imprisonment of active addiction may seem like an aspect of character we expect to "get" as soon as we are clean. Because of the chronic nature of the disease of addiction, however, and its bad effects on our lives, it often takes experience and time in recovery to appreciate our freedom and the responsibility that comes with it.

Freedom means knowing that even when we are in a circumstance where our choices are limited, we remain free to choose our attitude and response. Freedom means being responsible for consciously choosing *not* to act even when others expect and pressure us to do so. Freedom means being responsible for our actions, knowing we are as responsible for the questions we ask as we are for the answers we give in any situation.

When the Nazis imprisoned millions because they were considered racially inferior, it appeared all freedoms had been taken from those imprisoned. In fact, many of those imprisoned recognized and made choices that most people could not or would not see. Viktor E. Frankl wrote describing his choices as a prisoner, *"…everything can be taken from a man but one thing: the last of the human freedoms—to choose one's attitude in any given set of circumstances, to choose one's own way."****

MEDITATIVE THOUGHT

WHEN I AM ONLY FREE TO CHOOSE MY ATTITUDE, HELP ME REMEMBER THAT I HAVE THIS FREEDOM. WHEN MY CHOICES ARE LESS LIMITED, HELP ME FULLY EXERCISE MY FREEDOM FOR THE IMPROVEMENT OF MY OWN LIFE AND THE LIVES OF OTHERS.

Generous

Showing a readiness to give more of something,
especially money, than is strictly necessary or expected;
showing kindness toward others.

Oxford Dictionary of English*

• • •

"Do all the good you can,
By all the means you can,
In all the ways you can,
In all the places you can,
At all the times you can,
To all the people you can,
As long as ever you can."
John Wesley

Generosity was alien to most of us in active addiction. As we grow in recovery, our opportunities to be generous also grow. How we respond to these opportunities almost always depends on our spirituality. If we are spiritually fit, the opportunity to be generous will look like an opportunity to expand our potential and make connections with others. When we live in a diminished spiritual condition, we only see what things cost and are blind to the value of how these things can enrich our lives.

By permission of Oxford University Press. © 1998, 1999, 2001, 2003 by Oxford University Press.

Being alive, clean, and able to be generous are gifts that have been given to us in recovery. Guarding those resources, rather than sharing them, is the quickest and easiest way to lose them. When we are presented with the opportunity to be generous, our first reaction should be one of gratitude that we have anything worthwhile to give, followed by awareness that whatever we share we get to keep.

Sometimes being generous means giving our time to help someone else. Other times, generosity involves sharing some resource we have. Generosity always involves giving freely and without condition.

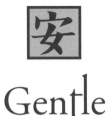

Gentle

Having or showing a mild, kind,
or tender temperament or character.
Oxford Dictionary of English*

• • •

"THAW WITH HIS GENTLE PERSUASION
IS MORE POWERFUL THAN THOR WITH HIS HAMMER.
THE ONE MELTS, THE OTHER BUT BREAKS IN PIECES."

HENRY DAVID THOREAU

In active addiction, there was little about us or our lives that could be described as gentle. In recovery, gentleness is not something we usually seek out. After admitting we were powerless, being gentle often seemed like one more way to be weak.

Our culture values strength and independence. We make movies, write books, and produce television programs that show strength, power, and oppression as ideals. We seldom consider how much real strength is required to be gentle. In truth, it takes more strength of character and self to sit quietly with someone in pain than it does to blow up something or hit someone.

Sitting with someone in pain, when all you have to offer is the comfort of your presence, requires that you acknowledge and accept everyone, including you, may have to one day face the same pain. It requires real courage to see that potential and remain present. Being gentle requires us to use our time, commitment, and humanness, rather than force or power, to accomplish our goals. Gentleness demands from us the time needed to understand and reach out to another. It makes us and those we interact with more human. Force and power make us and those we seek to change or defeat into objects, lessening our humanness.

Giving

Provide (love or other
emotional support) to.
*Oxford Dictionary of English**

• • •

"TO HAVE AND NOT TO GIVE
IS OFTEN WORSE THAN TO STEAL."

MARIE VON EBNER-ESCHENBACH

All of us, at some point, have given something to someone. Maybe we even gave to others during our active addiction. Most of us probably have packed up things we no longer want, need, or use to give to people or organizations. We are just as likely to have been moved by a desire to clean out our closets or our garages as the desire to give to someone else. This type of giving is instrumental giving and not the giving of character.

The giving of character refers to selfless generosity of spirit—the transfer of something or some quality that costs us something. When we specify that the giving "costs us," we're not referring to money. The cost of giving may be time or extra patience and compassion. This kind of giving often does not involve things. It is our motivation and the effects of our giving that matters.

When we give of our time, our resources, and our lives to enrich the life of another or to make the world a better place, we participate in the giving of character.

MEDITATIVE THOUGHT

HELP ME GIVE FREELY
FROM THE RESOURCES I CONSIDER VALUABLE IN MY LIFE.
AS I DO, MAKE ME AWARE OF THE BENEFITS OF THAT GIVING
TO OTHERS, THE WORLD, AND MYSELF.

Grateful

Feeling or showing an appreciation
for something done or received.

*Oxford Dictionary of English**

• • •

"IF THE ONLY PRAYER YOU SAY
IN YOUR LIFE IS "THANK YOU,"
THAT WOULD SUFFICE."

MEISTER ECKHART

Gratitude of character starts with a profound, often reverent appreciation of what we have been given. It extends to the action we take to honor that feeling. Sometimes this is feeling grateful to be clean and in recovery and getting out of a warm bed on a cold night to go on a twelve-step call. Sometimes it involves planning to honor a special day for someone we love; sometimes it is appreciating and acting to show the spontaneous generosity of spirit the program of recovery gives us.

The feeling of gratitude often is not visible to others. This feeling may be mistaken for something else; so it is important to share with others the depth of the gratitude that motivated us. In doing this, we humbly acknowledge the unearned gifts we've been given in recovery, as well as the gifts we have worked for and that provide an example of gratitude in action.

When we share our feeling of gratitude with another, it is important we connect the dots between our recovery, the gifts we've received, our feelings, thoughts, choices, and the consequences of our actions. This helps us take inventory to look for motives other than showing gratitude, which may creep into these situations. By doing this, we provide a living example of all recovery has to offer.

Hardworking

Tending to work with energy and commitment; diligent.
*Oxford Dictionary of English**

• • •

"HE HAS ACHIEVED SUCCESS WHO HAS LIVED WELL,
LAUGHED OFTEN, AND LOVED MUCH; WHO HAS ENJOYED
THE TRUST OF PURE WOMEN, THE RESPECT OF INTELLIGENT MEN,
AND THE LOVE OF SMALL CHILDREN; WHO HAS FILLED HIS NICHE,
AND ACCOMPLISHED HIS TASK; WHO HAS LEFT THE WORLD
BETTER THAN HE FOUND IT, WHETHER BY AN IMPROVED POPPY,
A PERFECT POEM, OR A RESCUED SOUL; WHO HAS NEVER
LACKED APPRECIATION OF EARTH'S BEAUTY, OR FAILED TO EXPRESS IT;
WHO HAS ALWAYS LOOKED FOR THE BEST IN OTHERS,
AND GIVEN THEM THE BEST HE HAD; WHOSE LIFE WAS AN INSPIRATION;
WHOSE MEMORY A BENEDICTION."

BESSIE ANDERSON STANLEY (PRIZE-WINNING DEFINITION OF *SUCCESS* IN A CONTEST
SPONSORED BY *BROWN BOOK OF BOSTON MAGAZINE,* 1904)

In active addiction, working hard was something we avoided. When we did work hard, it was usually in plotting and scheming to service our disease. In recovery, we learn the satisfaction of working smart and hard at the things important to us. To do this, we must consider our values and act in a way that respects those values. When we work hard at the important things to enrich our lives, our sense of satisfaction is often hard to describe.

We may find ourselves moved to tears by a sincere compliment from a friend or co-worker. We may enjoy the pervasive sense of well-being that accompanies our evaluation of our day at work. We may find the things that disturbed us in the morning are easier to accept later; or realize we need to make the effort to change those things if necessary.

Whether it's the quiet solitary satisfaction of a day well-lived or the sense of connection we get from having our work complimented, we see how working hard changes the quality of our life. As this happens, we become more able to pray, take action by working hard, and leave the results in the hands of our higher power. This adds to our sense of peace and well-being. We learn working hard, in balance with rest, self-care, and play, makes us happier and often makes other people happier with us.

MEDITATIVE THOUGHT

As I mindfully work hard
at those things I consider important,
help me gratefully acknowledge
how recovery has changed my life.

Honest

*Free of deceit; truthful and sincere;
morally correct or virtuous.*
Oxford Dictionary of English*

• • •

"HONESTY IS THE FIRST CHAPTER
OF THE BOOK OF WISDOM."

THOMAS JEFFERSON

Being honest was not a character asset for most of us during active addiction. When we got clean and began to work a recovery program, one of the first things we were told was that we would need to be honest, open-minded, and willing. If we were beaten by the disease of addiction and had surrendered to the process of recovery, being willing may have been relatively simple. If we accepted our ideas about life had not worked out well, being open-minded may have come relatively easy, too. However, when it comes to being honest, most of us have trouble even knowing where to begin. We may truly want to be honest, but still struggle with it. This is often because we have been dishonest with ourselves for so long that we have trouble distinguishing the truth from a lie. In other words, because we lied to ourselves about so many things those lies now seem real.

Coming to terms with being honest requires we work the steps with a sponsor. It requires a searching and fearless moral inventory. Our sponsor can help us see where we have deluded ourselves, where we have lied to excuse our behavior, and even where we have been too hard on ourselves. Once we can be honest with ourselves about our behavior and motives, we can start to be honest with others.

Often in our eagerness to share this newfound gift, we tend to use honesty like a weapon and share more than we are asked. When we do this, we cross the line from honest reflection to judging or imposing our view of the world. We must seek a healthy balance between honesty and tact, learning to be honest while respecting the rights of others to grow at their higher power's pace. We learn to share what is asked of us honestly and with love, rather than seeing ourselves as the guardians of truth.

MEDITATIVE THOUGHT

HELP ME BE AS HONEST AS I CAN.
HELP ME LEARN TO BE MORE HONEST
AS I LEARN TO BALANCE MY AWARENESS
WITH BEING LOVING AND RESPECTFUL OF OTHERS.

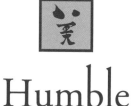

Humble

Having or showing a modest
or low estimate of one's importance.
*Oxford Dictionary of English**

• • •

"WHEN PRIDE COMES, THEN COMES DISGRACE,
BUT WITH HUMILITY COMES WISDOM."
THE BIBLE, PROVERBS 11:2

As using addicts, humility was not apparent in most of our lives. We often thought of ourselves as being less than others, while thinking only of ourselves. This frequently resulted in selfish, self-absorbed self-hatred. Other times in active addiction, we saw ourselves as better, smarter, and slicker than others. This usually resulted in self-important, self-absorbed isolation. No matter how we thought of ourselves, we usually were alone and unhappy.

In recovery, as we write steps with our sponsor, we gain a realistic picture of who we are—our good points, as well as our less attractive qualities. We begin to see how we are more similar to others than different. Our picture of who we are gains depth and clarity. With depth and clarity comes humility.

We start to see the ways we are different as characteristics, not evidence. If these differences are positive, we see these characteristics as opportunities to contribute.

We stop seeing them as attributes that make us better and begin to see them only as part of who we are. When the differences are not positive or helpful, we realize how these differences can make our lives harder.

When we accept less attractive characteristics, we gain the opportunity to seek freedom from them through the Twelve Steps, our relationship with our sponsor, and our higher power. When we can accept who we are, then we are humble. When we are humble, we are teachable and can grow.

Integrity

The quality of being honest and having strong moral principles;
the state of being whole and undivided;
the condition of being unified or sound in construction.

Oxford Dictionary of English*

• • •

"INTEGRITY WITHOUT KNOWLEDGE
IS WEAK AND USELESS,
AND KNOWLEDGE WITHOUT INTEGRITY
IS DANGEROUS AND DREADFUL."

SAMUEL JOHNSON

Often in active addiction, the rules we followed were those dictated to us by our disease. In the grip of addiction, even if we knew what our values were, we were powerless to live by them. In recovery, we are responsible for our choices and actions, and as we are restored to sanity, we become whole and sound. We develop the ability to examine and decide what

our values are, and we are given the freedom to live our lives guided by those values.

Integrity makes it possible for us to decide if the standards demanded of us are too low. It gives us the opportunity to choose to live by rules we develop for ourselves. Integrity also makes it possible for us to decide whether the standards demanded of us are too high to follow. Unlike the noncompliance or sneaky rule-breaking we did in active addiction, when we act with integrity in our recovery and refuse to adhere to the standards of others, we do so clearly, calmly, and directly.

We may decide we are unwilling to do what would make us more financially successful because it would cost too much of the family time we value. We may decide to change careers, or we may simply tell our boss that we are happy doing a good job at our present level and do not want to advance. We may decide a community culture that condones excluding some people for reasons we cannot respect, is not acceptable. This may mean moving, changing schools, or working to change the community in which we live.

Whatever we decide to do, when we do it from the integrity of our character, we can be sure we will continue to learn, grow, and change. We also can be sure our recovery will be enhanced as we practice integrity.

Interdependent

Mutual dependence with (not on)
others in a healthy, sustainable way.

Denise D. Crosson, Ph.D., RN, FNP-CS

• • •

"SUCH HELP AS WE CAN GIVE EACH OTHER
IN THIS WORLD IS A *DEBT* TO EACH OTHER;
AND THE MAN WHO PERCEIVES A SUPERIORITY
OR CAPACITY IN A SUBORDINATE,
AND NEITHER CONFESSES NOR ASSISTS IT,
IS NOT MERELY THE WITHHOLDER OF KINDNESS,
BUT THE COMMITTER OF INJURY."

JOHN RUSKIN

Interdependence was not possible in our lives in active addiction. We could not be counted on to behave in a consistent, healthy, interdependent manner when we were using, and we did not trust others enough to rely on them. We often were dependent on others for our basic needs and for things we were responsible for doing ourselves. We did this out of desperation, not trust.

Other times, we may have tried to do it all by ourselves and go it alone in a show of independence. We did this not from a place of responsibility, but usually out of bravado or because we damaged so many relationships there was no one left to help us. Either way, we ended up feeling alone and felt "one down" when we were dependent and "one up" when we were independent.

Interdependence becomes possible as we grow in recovery and become more reliable, trustworthy, trusting, and willing to accept help. As we learn to be responsible for our recovery while accepting help and support from others, we develop the ability to have peers. We learn that in the same relationship, often within the course of minutes or hours, we can both accept help and offer help. We learn the most helpful, appropriate response can and should depend on the circumstance—from surrender and acceptance to prayer and action. We learn to vary our approach and role in relationships based on recovery and reality rather than on the demands of our disease.

Interdependence helps keep our perspective while we stay "right sized." When we are interdependent we are never "one up" or "one down" from anyone. We may have more experience, knowledge, or wisdom than someone else, but we remember there are other circumstances where we had less and benefited from relying on others.

When we are interdependent we are open to the process of recovery and to whatever life offers or asks. We see ourselves as an important part of life, but no more or less important than anyone else.

Just

Based on or behaving according to what is
morally right and fair; (of treatment) deserved
or appropriate in the circumstances.

Oxford Dictionary of English*

• • •

"IF WE SHOULD DEAL OUT JUSTICE ONLY,
IN THIS WORLD, WHO WOULD ESCAPE?
NO, IT IS BETTER TO BE GENEROUS,
AND IN THE END MORE PROFITABLE,
FOR IT GAINS GRATITUDE FOR US, AND LOVE."

MARK TWAIN

What was morally right or fair was of little concern to many of us during our active addiction. We often were more interested in getting something for nothing. Many of us bring this same attitude into recovery. We may give it little thought or we may believe if we can get away with "something for nothing," then it's okay.

As we work the Twelve Steps, our awareness of the gap between our attitudes and actions and what is morally correct grows. If we truly embrace the principles of the steps, we become increasingly aware of this gap by taking a searching and fearless moral inventory. How, after years of trying to get over, do we begin to behave in a just manner?

The simplest answer is that we start from where we are.

If we catch ourselves in a lie as we are telling it, we own up to it and tell the truth. If we become aware of the unjustness of our actions after the fact, we check with our sponsor and take whatever action is needed to amend the situation. If we treat someone unfairly, we make amends.

We must look at the circumstances, examine our actions, and determine the consequences of those actions. Then we take whatever actions are needed to help us behave correctly in the future.

Kind

Having or showing a friendly,
generous, and considerate nature.

Oxford Dictionary of English*

• • •

"KINDNESS IS IN OUR POWER,
EVEN WHEN FONDNESS IS NOT."

SAMUEL JOHNSON

Kindness is another character trait often thought of as old-fashioned or as a soft virtue. Being kind requires we bring other character traits to bear. In order to be kind, we must have the ability to notice, consider, and act on what would be helpful and welcome by another. We must be self- and other-aware, and we must be capable of selflessness and generosity.

Sometimes kindness is a sincere, well-timed smile of support. Other times, it requires our effort to be present and silent when words are not adequate or it asks us to empathize with or support another.

Our lives are full of opportunities to be kind. How often and how well we respond to these opportunities will influence the quality of our own lives and the lives of those around us. We do not have to know someone to be kind. We may be kind by allowing another driver out of a tight intersection. We may be kind to a tired mother with a cranky child by letting her go ahead of us in line at the grocery store. We may be kind to our children by attending more to their successes than their failures. We may be kind to our spouse by simply letting an unintended slight pass without comment. Whether we ever see a response or whether the response is immediate or delayed, there is a benefit to kindness in our lives and in the lives of others.

Loving

Feeling or showing love or great care.
Oxford Dictionary of English*

• • •

"AS LOVE WITHOUT ESTEEM IS CAPRICIOUS AND VOLATILE;
ESTEEM WITHOUT LOVE IS LANGUID AND COLD."

JONATHAN SWIFT

Being loving is one of the most misunderstood of all character traits. The confusion is the belief that love is simply a feeling and "being in love" is the desired goal or condition. In fact, being in love is usually infatuation, which is often more about seeing what we want to see in another and loving that illusion.

Love is about seeing people or ideals for what they actually are and embracing and supporting that reality. Love is expressed differently, but is the same across different relationships. How we *show* love to our partner will be different than with our friends or children; however, the basic nature is the same.

Love is as simple, yet demanding, as seeing the parts of our loved ones' personalities that are not as we would like them to be and accepting and loving them as whole people without having to make excuses or redecorate the reality of who they are. Love often is confused for a bartering system. Love does not demand, "If you love me, do this," or "If you *really* loved me you would not do that." Love is based on connection at its most whole and most spiritual level.

Love, when truly felt and practiced, seldom brings our needs in conflict with the needs of our loved ones. In love, the importance of mutual needs is greater than individual needs. On the rare occasion when mutual and individual needs conflict, being loving requires that we put our loved one's interests ahead of our own. In doing so, we find that our mutual good is far more important and fulfilling than our individual desires.

As we practice this principle and become more loving, we are better able to receive love in return. This is not infatuation-type love. It is the nurturing type of caring relationship in which we are connected to others in ways that expand and add to who we are and who we will be.

In order to love we must have someone to love. We are unable to feel or express love, other than self-love, in a vacuum. Love requires us to be willing to be vulnerable, seen, heard, and known for who we are and that we have the strength and willingness to see, hear, and know another for who he or she is.

MEDITATIVE THOUGHT

HELP ME LIVE AS IF SHOWING LOVE IS THE MOST IMPORTANT THING I WILL DO. HELP ME SHOW LOVE TO MYSELF AND OTHERS. LET ME ENJOY THE SENSE OF STRENGTH AND COMMITMENT THAT FLOWS FROM BEING VULNERABLE TO THE CONNECTION WITH OTHERS.

Mature

(Especially of a young person) having reached a stage
of mental or emotional development characteristic of an adult;
(of thought or planning) careful and thorough.

Oxford Dictionary of English*

• • •

"THE GOOD OF MAN IS THE ACTIVE EXERCISE OF HIS
SOUL'S FACULTIES IN CONFORMITY WITH EXCELLENCE OR VIRTUE…
MOREOVER THIS ACTIVITY MUST OCCUPY A COMPLETE LIFETIME;
FOR ONE SWALLOW DOES NOT MAKE SPRING, NOR DOES ONE FINE DAY;
AND SIMILARLY ONE DAY OR A BRIEF PERIOD OF HAPPINESS
DOES NOT MAKE A MAN SUPREMELY BLESSED AND HAPPY."

ARISTOTLE

Maturity can always be avoided in life. In active addiction, we often placed other priorities ahead of attention to our lives and the efforts to learn from our mistakes that are required for maturation. As a result, many of us enter recovery less mature than our chronological age. This immaturity is not always apparent.

If we have been superficially compliant with the world's expectations of us while in active addiction, our lives and maturity might appear less affected at first glance. We may have tangible evidence of maturity, such as intact families, jobs, houses, and cars. Sometimes we have retained these adult things by our own efforts, sometimes by the efforts of our partners and families. But in the end, having a job and owning things does not mean we are mature adults; it means we have a job and tangible stuff.

In recovery we learn being mature means taking responsibility for our lives—physically, financially, emotionally, and spiritually. On a practical and financial level, it is relatively easy to see if we are responsible. In recovery, to evaluate our emotional, spiritual, and relational maturity, we must write the steps and seek and accept the guidance and help of our sponsor. Without the help given us through writing, practicing, and being sponsored on the steps, we can lose our ability to see ourselves clearly and become lost in rationalization and justification.

With help, however, we are free to grow and change into mature, whole people free from the negative drain of our disease. When we are mature, we become better able to survive our feelings. We know even when we feel bad we are more than what we feel and that our feelings will eventually change. Knowing this gives us the opportunity to be and act as who we are rather than react in an effort to change how we feel.

The advantages of maturity are many, including comfort in our own skin, freedom from a life run entirely by our feelings and our desire to change them, the ability to trust ourselves, and the ability to be trusted by others.

Open-minded

Willing to consider new ideas; unprejudiced.

Oxford Dictionary of English*

• • •

"WHAT WE HAVE TO DO IS TO BE FOR EVER CURIOUSLY TESTING
NEW OPINIONS AND COURTING NEW IMPRESSIONS."

WALTER PATER

People often confuse being open-minded with not having a firm position. In fact, having firm convictions, based on criteria we have decided are important to us, is almost a requirement of being open-minded. Being open-minded means listening attentively and respectfully to the position of another. It does not require we fully understand, agree, or support the position. Almost invariably, we find the more certain we are of our own position, the less we need to make someone with a different position wrong.

If we are clear and certain about what we believe, and have looked at how we might see things differently, as well as consciously considered that we may be wrong, chances are we probably won't feel so defensive or combative when others disagree with us. We won't feel pressure to convince them of the rightness of our view; rather, we simply know it is right for us in this time, place, and circumstance.

When we are less certain of our view, but are able to be open-minded, we can enjoy spirited dialogue with others. Not only do we often enjoy it, but we examine it for ways it can help us clarify our own beliefs and thoughts. Usually, the more confusion and less certainty we have about a matter, the more vigorous our argument tends to be for "my position." When we are able to do this with an open mind, it can be amazing what we learn about others, the world, and ourselves. The dialogue of searching almost always results in our feeling more connected to the world and to those to whom we listen.

When we are unwilling to consider we could be wrong or when a "position" is so sacred it feels heretical to question it, we place ourselves on dangerous ground. Large or important ideas should be subject to the same scrutiny and consideration as small, less important ones. When we cannot scrutinize a position, chances are we cannot be open-minded about it. Seeking dialogue in this circumstance often results in argument and the attempt to oppress others whose views are different than our own since considering the possibility we might be wrong is too threatening to allow an open mind.

MEDITATIVE THOUGHT

MANY OF THE LESSONS AND KNOWLEDGE AVAILABLE IN LIFE DO NOT COME WITH NEAT LABELS, BUT CAN BE APPLIED IN AREAS FAR DIFFERENT THAN WHERE WE LEARN THEM. HELP ME BE OPEN-MINDED, TO LEARN AND USE THE LESSONS IN MY LIFE WHEREVER THEY WORK TO HELP OTHERS, THE WORLD, AND ME. HELP ME CELEBRATE BEING WRONG FOR THE LESSONS IT PROVIDES AS I CELEBRATE BEING RIGHT.

Optimistic

Hopeful and confident about the future.

*Oxford Dictionary of English**

• • •

"I ALWAYS PREFER TO BELIEVE THE BEST OF EVERYBODY,
IT SAVES SO MUCH TROUBLE."

RUDYARD KIPLING

The approach recommended by Rudyard Kipling is often seen as naïve. Today it seems that movies, books, and everyday life place much value on getting the best of others before they have a chance to take advantage of us. This outlook means we expect the worst from nearly everyone.

Our lives in active addiction undoubtedly supported this suspicious and pessimistic view. In recovery, however, we need to understand how our behavior and choices affect how we are treated by others. In recovery, if we come to believe we are guided and protected by our higher power, then even relationships that disappoint us offer lessons and opportunities for growth.

In recovery, we try to believe the best of everyone. That way we have a more relaxed and open life; a life in which we are better able to see things as they are rather than as we fear they might be. When people disappoint us by not living up to our expectations, we still have the peace and freedom of knowing their choices were not negatively influenced by our view of them. Relaxation and openness allows us to live more mindfully and effectively as the person we want to be.

An optimistic belief in others leaves them free to be who they are without our attempting to control them or without us personalizing their behavior.

MEDITATIVE THOUGHT

As I live in today,
help me see the world and my life optimistically.
Help me enjoy the peace and freedom
of seeing others in the best possible light.

Patient

Able to accept or tolerate delays, problems, or suffering
without becoming annoyed or anxious.

Oxford Dictionary of English*

• • •

"OUR PATIENCE WILL ACHIEVE MORE THAN OUR FORCE."

EDMUND BURKE

Patience was not a prominent attribute for many of us while in active addiction. We may have waited what seemed like endless hours for others to bring us drugs, but we didn't do it patiently. We did it because we could see no choice other than to do what our disease required of us.

Even in early recovery the options and choices available to us may seem astounding compared with our lives when we were using. Despite the freedom recovery brings us, patience usually is not natural or easy for us. We often want what we want "right now." Some of this is a natural desire to make a life worth living in the face of the time we wasted in active addiction. Some of this is an attempt to get it all, right this minute, which is just another way our disease is trying to run our lives.

As we work a program of recovery we start to develop faith in the program and the people who help us stay clean. As our faith grows and we continue to work the program, we develop a sense of being guided and protected. We may notice circumstances and events often work out by accident better than what we could have planned or controlled. We may notice that when we don't know what to do next, if we ask for help and wait, the answer becomes clear. When we have this attitude of acceptance and gratitude for guidance, it becomes easier to wait patiently for the future to unfold. We feel less pressure to rush to conclusions and more willing to wait to see what happens.

Practicing patience in recovery is not saying the first thing that pops into our head. It is the effort we make to be even-tempered. Sometimes practicing patience is avoiding an urgently felt need to fix ourselves with something external in order to change how we feel.

The rewards of patience are many and far-reaching, including calm acceptance of our powerlessness, more energy to devote to the things that are our responsibility, relationships that are more peaceful and harmonious, life without the artificial drama of crisis-to-crisis living, and an internalized sense of access to the power we need to live in recovery through the Twelve Steps.

MEDITATIVE THOUGHT

LET ME WORK A PROGRAM OF RECOVERY, PRAY, MEDITATE,
AND APPROACH ALL THAT I DO WITH PATIENCE.
HELP ME SEE THAT THE LONG VIEW OF LIFE IS MORE SATISFYING
THAN THE MINUTE-TO-MINUTE REPLAY.

Practical

Of or concerned with actually doing or use of something
rather than with theory and ideas; (of an idea, plan, or method)
likely to succeed or be effective in real circumstances; feasible;
suitable for a particular purpose; (of a person) sensible and realistic
in their approach to a situation or problem.

*Oxford Dictionary of English**

• • •

"Never be completely idle, but either reading,
or writing, or praying, or meditating,
or some useful work for the common good."

Thomas á Kempis

Few relate practicality to character and it is frequently underrated as a skill or ability. Being practical, however, requires one to have some skill with a number of other character assets such as discernment, patience, open-mindedness, alertness, altruism, decisiveness, and courage.

Being practical requires we maintain a balance between thinking and plodding along thoughtlessly. It means using all our assets to find solutions to problems or situations.

A course of action may be easy or possible, but if it conflicts with our values it is not practical. Another course of action may be consistent with our values, but impossible to do. For example, we may be deeply disturbed by the fact that there are people in the world who are hungry. We may want to change this fact, but we don't have the resources to fund the solution.

Practicality allows us to understand what we can possibly and effectively change. It lets us consider what we can change in our own lives that will support greater change in this area. Eating everything on our plates, to our own detriment or distaste, will not make any practical difference to others who are hungry. Even if doing so is consistent with a value we have about not being wasteful, it's not effective, and so it isn't practical. In contrast, volunteering or donating groceries to a soup kitchen in our community is consistent with our value of generosity and not wasting and is effective since it results in actually feeding hungry people, making it a low-key, but practical solution to our concern.

Being practical is not the same as settling for the fastest, closest, or easiest solution or approach. It requires that we seek and try the most functional solution or approach. When we do this, being practical enhances our daily and spiritual life.

MEDITATIVE THOUGHT

HELP ME APPROACH LIFE WITH THE PRACTICALITY OF CHARACTER.
HELP ME FIND BALANCE BETWEEN
THE POSSIBILITY OF IMAGINATION AND IDEALISM
AND THE GRAVITATIONAL PULL
OF THE PRESSURES OF DAILY LIFE AND REALISM.

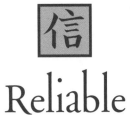

Reliable

Consistently good in quality or performance;
able to be trusted.

Oxford Dictionary of English*

• • •

"THE FRIEND OF MY ADVERSITY I SHALL ALWAYS CHERISH THE MOST.
I CAN BETTER TRUST THOSE WHO HELPED
TO RELIEVE THE GLOOM OF MY DARK HOURS
THAN THOSE WHO ARE SO READY TO ENJOY WITH ME
THE SUNSHINE OF MY PROSPERITY."

ULYSSES S. GRANT

When we were in active addiction, no sane person would have relied on most of us. We weren't consistent in our actions or attitudes. We usually only acted on whatever we needed to do next in order to get or use drugs. In active addiction, our lives often were too complicated by our disease to allow us to be reliable.

In recovery, we learn to simplify our lives. We learn we cannot split life between recovery and other competing demands. We learn to put our recovery ahead of all else. By doing this we can prioritize and later add other demands. As we do this, reliability becomes part of our character and part of who we are.

When reliability is part of our character, we perform well and act consistently. The reliability of character means we support good ideas even when these ideas are offered by people who aren't friends or allies. It also means we don't support ideas inconsistent with our values even when offered by someone we respect or love.

Being reliable means people can count on us to do what we say we will do even if we don't feel like it. Being reliable also means we recognize and expend effort to meet our duties to ourselves even if it makes us look selfish.

Being reliable makes us trustworthy, which simplifies our lives, puts us at peace, and helps us feel good about our lives. Being reliable makes us feel whole, strong, and safe—even in the face of risk or danger.

Respectful

Feeling or showing deference and respect.
Oxford Dictionary of English*

• • •

"SELF-RESPECT—THAT CORNER-STONE OF ALL VIRTUE."

SIR JOHN HERSCHEL

Our ability to feel and show respect was severely affected in active addiction. In recovery, we are free to make choices about who and what we respect, as well as how to show the respect we feel.

We may want to consider whether we believe respect is earned by others or whether we believe all people are inherently worthy of respect. We also might want to consider whether we respect all socially sanctioned institutions or whether we will feel and show respect only for those institutions that are consistent with our own values. These are questions to which there are no right or wrong answers. Nevertheless, it is important we answer them honestly, for these answers and how we implement them in our lives can affect the quality of our lives and our sense of well-being.

Respect, self-respect, and dignity are intimately related. How we see others and ourselves will guide how we treat others and ourselves. If we believe we deserve respect, but don't extend that same respect to others, our sense of self-worth will likely suffer. If we believe respect is something that must be earned and then give it unearned to those we like, but withhold it from those we do not like, we will not be living in our values. If we claim to respect someone yet violate his or her dignity, we again are living a lie.

Only by asking and answering the questions about to whom, what, and/or how we show respect can we gain the full measure of freedom and peace that is available to us in recovery.

MEDITATIVE THOUGHT

HELP ME ASK, AND THEN ANSWER HONESTLY,
THE QUESTIONS I NEED TO CONSIDER
ABOUT RESPECTING MYSELF AND OTHERS.
HELP ME FEEL AND SHOW GRATITUDE FOR THE FREEDOM AND PEACE
THAT COME TO ME AS A RESULT OF THIS WORK.

Responsible

Having an obligation to do something,
or having control over or care for someone,
as part of one's job or role.
Oxford Dictionary of English*

• • •

"LET EVERYONE SWEEP IN FRONT OF HIS OWN DOOR,
AND THE WHOLE WORLD WILL BE CLEAN."
JOHANN WOLFGANG VON GOETHE

Being responsible is a very demanding character asset. It requires that we know ourselves and own our choices and the consequences of those choices. Being responsible means knowing what things in life are in our control and focusing our attention on those things.

Often, in active addiction, we flip-flopped between making outrageous excuses for inexcusable behavior and taking responsibility for our behavior, while feeling guilty for things that were out of our control. In recovery, we learn to tell the difference between these things. We can learn about being responsible by listening with an open mind to our sponsors, other recovering friends, and family. We do our best to seek and consider their experience, strength, and hope.

At times it may be difficult to recognize we are making a choice. We may try to avoid responsibility by delaying a decision until we have fewer and fewer options and then tell ourselves, "If only I'd known then what I know now, I could have...." We may try to get others to decide for us so we can hold them responsible if our choice does not work out. These actions may give us an alibi or excuse, but they seldom make our lives better. Failing to notice or denying we have a choice is one of the risks of not knowing ourselves and not paying attention to our world. To be responsible we must know who we are and what we are doing, as well as where we fit in the world. Then we must be able to fearlessly own the choices we make, even when they don't work out as we'd like. When we are responsible we find we need to explain or apologize less. Being responsible also means we will have more peace in our lives as we have less to fear or regret.

MEDITATIVE THOUGHT

HELP ME ACT RESPONSIBLY IN ALL I DO.
HELP ME NOTICE THE PEACE AND FREEDOM
FROM FEAR AND REGRET
THAT FLOWS FROM MY RESPONSIBILITY.

Self-discipline

The ability to control one's feelings
and overcome one's weaknesses.

Oxford Dictionary of English*

• • •

"IT IS BETTER TO CONQUER YOURSELF
THAN TO WIN A THOUSAND BATTLES.
THEN THE VICTORY IS YOURS.
IT CANNOT BE TAKEN FROM YOU,
NOT BY ANGELS OR BY DEMONS, HEAVEN OR HELL."

SIDDHARTHA BUDDHA

One of the things the disease of addiction robbed us of was the ability to practice self-discipline. Whatever self-discipline we might have had early in life was so subverted and consumed by our disease that it was unrecognizable in most of us at the end of active addiction. Most of us answered only to the call and demands of our disease—disciplining ourselves to do whatever we needed to get the next drug or get out of whatever mess we had made while using.

In recovery, we begin to learn the self-discipline required to stay clean. We learn to plan our days around self-care, such as attending meetings; calling our sponsors; getting adequate rest, exercise, and food; maintaining balance between recovery, family, and friends; and going to work. As we learn this day-to-day self-discipline, we build the foundation needed to develop control in other areas. Self-discipline in our emotional, spiritual, and relational affairs is just as important, but harder to grasp. This is the self-discipline of character.

The self-discipline of character is too often confused with being hard on ourselves. In truth, self-discipline is the easiest way to be gentle with ourselves and the easiest way to find freedom from self. Self-discipline of character lets us take responsibility to create the kind of structure for our lives that gives us the freedom to do nearly anything we want. Self-discipline gives us the experience and wisdom to choose what we want to do and to do it wisely. Self-discipline is passing up the opportunity for instant gratification in favor of something more important that requires more time or effort.

Self-discipline requires we know ourselves and accept responsibility for our actions. Then we can see and accept the connection between our choices and the consequences of those choices. When we do this, we are free from trying to gain approval from others. When we are self-disciplined, we can enjoy the relationships in our lives because we are not dependent on others for structure or wisdom.

When we are self-disciplined, we find the standards we set for ourselves in recovery are higher than those required of us by others.

MEDITATIVE THOUGHT

HELP ME CREATE THE INTERNAL AND EXTERNAL STRUCTURE
I NEED TO BE SELF-DISCIPLINED.
HELP ME APPRECIATE THIS SELF-DISCIPLINE
AS A WAY TO BE GENTLE WITH MYSELF
AND SUPPORT MY FREEDOM.

Selfless

Concerned more with the needs and wishes of others
than with one's own; unselfish.

*Oxford Dictionary of English**

• • •

"THE DEED IS ALL, THE GLORY NOTHING."

JOHANN WOLFGANG VON GOETHE

In active addiction, most of us were concerned only with those things that enabled us to get and use drugs. Selflessness in recovery requires we act as if our wishes and needs are not the most important thing in the world. A recovering addict, Sydney R, once revealed that in our efforts to be selfless, we should ask ourselves, "What would a loving God have me do?" She explained how important it is to not only ask this, but also to do our best to live as if that question were the most important question in the world.

Sydney demonstrated this in an incident in which she was involved with a health care worker. She was recovering from a difficult illness and was sick and tired most of the day. The effort of daily living took a lot out of her as she worked on healing.

One day, while on a health-related errand, Sydney was mistreated by someone who owed her a duty of attention and professionalism. Sydney calmly responded to his mistreatment and politely told him that she could appreciate what a difficult job he had and that she could not imagine what it took to do it. Then, she told him how she felt and what she needed.

She framed her feelings and needs in terms of asking for his help. As she spoke, she maintained calm, steady, and non-threatening eye contact with him and wore a genuine, but tired smile. When she finished speaking he was silent for a moment, and then said, "Look, I'm really sorry. I guess I was being pretty awful to you. You should probably complain about me."

Sydney said nothing and sat very still. She did not say "Oh that's okay, don't worry about it." She did not say "That's right, you're a jerk." She just sat there and said nothing for a while, and then finally said "I don't want to complain. I just want to get this over with as painlessly as possible for both of us." Because of her behavior, this person really heard what she said, and he could see that she meant it. He looked both relieved and grateful, and then did exactly what she asked him to do—attentively and professionally.

Afterward, Sydney explained: "Everybody has bad days. Everybody fails to show up as who they'd like to be sometimes. What you have to ask yourself is what would a loving God have me do? If you can take the time to ask and answer that question, and then do whatever the answer is, you never have to act like a selfish, insensitive person."

This example shows how Sydney was able to practice selfless behavior with the health worker who mistreated her. She came from a place of love and at the same time she wanted very badly to never be like the other person had been with her. Being him, as he had been before their conversation, was its own punishment. As a recovering person, we all have responsibility for our actions, separate from someone else's behavior.

Sensitive

Quick to detect or respond to slight changes, signals, or influences; having or displaying a quick and delicate appreciation of others' feelings.

Oxford Dictionary of English*

• • •

"WE FEEL OUR GOOD AND OUR BAD FORTUNE SOLELY IN PROPORTION TO OUR SELF-LOVE."

FRANÇOIS, DUC DE LA ROCHEFOUCAULD

We often tried to numb our sensitivity through drugs in active addiction, while without drugs we were probably too sensitive. In recovery, we may try to use other things to avoid being sensitive such as burying ourselves in work, relationships, sex, food, or gambling. These things may work temporarily to numb us, but they come with many of the same costs as drug use.

In recovery, as we learn to trust the process and work the Twelve Steps, we develop greater balance with sensitivity. We come to know ourselves and feel safer in the world, and some of our over-sensitivity is relieved. As we become more sensitive we find we can survive feelings without being numb, and our appreciation of the benefits of sensitivity grows.

Sensitivity requires honesty, courage, patience, attention, and presence. Being sensitive can be sitting quietly and attending to how we feel in the presence of another. Other times sensitivity requires more active attention such as choosing between follow-up or keeping still with a vague, ill-defined feeling about something until we have more clarity.

When we are sensitive we become better at detecting and responding to subtle changes that simplify, expand, and enrich our lives. Sensitivity helps us understand and respond appropriately and helpfully to the world. Sensitivity helps make us better able to participate in our recovery. It also helps to make us better friends, partners, employees, supervisors, sponsors, sponsees, or family members. Sensitivity of character cannot fail to affect and enrich all of our relationships.

MEDITATIVE THOUGHT

HELP ME EMBRACE SENSITIVITY WITH THE CALM ASSURANCE
THAT I WILL SURVIVE MY FEELINGS.
HELP ME APPRECIATE THE WAYS IN WHICH MY SENSITIVITY
ENRICHES AND EXPANDS MY LIFE AND RELATIONSHIPS.

Sincere

Free from pretense or deceit; proceeding from genuine feelings;
(of a person) saying what they genuinely feel or believe;
not dishonest or hypocritical.

Oxford Dictionary of English*

• • •

"SINCERITY AND TRUTH ARE THE BASIS OF EVERY VIRTUE."

CONFUCIUS

To many, sincerity may pale as a character asset when compared with discernment, courage, wisdom, or honesty. Sincerity, however, requires we possess all of these assets. To be sincere, we must have the wisdom and discernment to know others, our world, and ourselves, coupled with the courage and honesty to express what we know.

Sincerity requires thoughtful attention to what we believe, feel, or see before we speak or act, and we do it without deceit or pretense.

We seldom had the time or resources to be sincere when we were using. That was due to our untreated disease. Active addiction was about changing our perception of reality with drugs or using other people, places, or things instead of living with reality.

When we use drugs we run from ourselves and reality. Most of us run because we believe we are flawed and no one, including ourselves, could or should love us. The essence of insincerity is our belief that people, including ourselves, cannot be trusted and the world is a dangerous place. We believe being genuine and keeping our hearts open makes us vulnerable. From this perspective we only see others and the world in terms of what we want from them. This robs us of the opportunity to connect on a spiritual and emotional level.

As we begin to trust the process of recovery, we learn to work and embrace the principles embodied in the Twelve Steps. When we work the steps, we realize we are neither as awful nor as perfect as we saw ourselves in active addiction. This usually leads to awareness that the world is neither as awful nor as perfect as we imagined.

We learn to accept ourselves as we work toward growth and change. We learn about our emotional and spiritual strengths and about the resources available to us from our higher power, sponsor, and friends. We learn to accept others and the world as they are. When we do this, we accept the uncertainty of life with grace, and we are empowered to feel strong and capable even as we acknowledge our vulnerability.

By being sincere we have the ability to make connections with others, our higher power, and the world. In order to live in the present, we must be sincere. In order to remain in recovery, we must live in the present.

SINCERITY IS ESSENTIAL TO MY RECOVERY.
WITH IT, I AM CAPABLE OF KNOWING AND EMBRACING REALITY.
HELP ME LIVE IN SINCERITY AND POSSIBILITY.

Spiritual

Relating to or affecting the human spirit or soul
as opposed to material or physical things;
having a relationship based on a profound level of
mental or emotional communion.

Oxford Dictionary of English*

• • •

"LET US LOVE, NOT IN WORD OR SPEECH,
BUT IN TRUTH AND ACTION."

THE BIBLE, 1 JOHN 3:18

We often separate things into categories and concepts so we are better able to talk about them. This does not mean these things are truly separate.

Instructors discuss the respiratory system as a separate topic in the study of anatomy. This is done to help students understand how the respiratory system works with the rest of our bodies. The respiratory system does not exist as a separate entity, only as part of our bodies.

Our intellect, emotions, thoughts, actions, and relationships join together to form the essence and expression of our spirit. Our spirit is the product of all of the parts of our life. The spirit is the whole person; the intellect forms the central nervous system; emotions are the heart and gut, and actions make up the muscles and bones. While not a perfect analogy, it offers an example of the process of change we experience when we embrace recovery.

In recovery, we have the opportunity to consciously examine all the parts of our spirits through the Twelve Steps. Each step addresses a separate part so that we can better understand the whole.

The First Step teaches powerlessness. It shows us how small we are compared to the disease of addiction. Step One is not about helplessness, but rather becoming aware of and accepting what we can and cannot change. This awareness is necessary for humility and gives us a sense of place in the world.

We learn about faith and hope in the Second Step and how a benign power—neither of our making nor under our control—can restore us to sanity. The process of coming to believe helps us develop optimism about our place in the world. This step reminds us of the connection we must seek to live with our powerlessness without being controlled by it.

The Third Step shows us how to seek that connection through the surrender of what is not ours to control and take responsibility for the things we do control. If we are to learn about commitment, responsibility, and self-discipline, we need to do our best to embrace the principles embodied in this step.

In the Fourth Step, we review what we have done with the spirits given to us at birth and to examine how well our spirits have worked for us. Step Four helps us confront what we have done in life and what we believe and value. It also shows us when, how, and sometimes why we have failed to honor what we believe and value and what that has cost us. Without this vital inventory, we will not come to know our spirits, choices, and the consequences of our choices.

We learn about trust, faith, and humility in the Fifth Step. Sharing on such an intimate level as the Fifth Step encourages us to do so, we see that others can be trusted and how they relate to and complement our lives. We also see how we failed to honor the gift of spirit and recovery in the past.

[continued on page 106]

Willingness is a major component of the Sixth Step and teaches us to look closely at the patterns in our lives. As we continue with the recovery process, we do our best to keep an open mind and examine how we respond to the world around us. We do the work that is ours to do and learn to seek the help we need to be relieved of what hinders our recovery.

In the Seventh Step, we ask for and stay open to getting what we need. It shows us there are some things in life that are not ours to control or fix. Step Seven teaches us that we cannot work on ourselves, but rather we can only ask our higher power and the program to work on us. This is not to say we just sit around and wait to be changed, but rather we do the work necessary to change. Exactly how and when we change is up to our higher power.

The Eighth Step shows us that we have a responsibility for what we do to others when we try to get what we need or want in a way that violates our values and the values of others. In this step, we focus on our willingness to change and face the harm we caused directly or indirectly.

While we are not always able to amend the pain and harm we may have caused, in the Ninth Step we are empowered to offer restitution for some of the destruction. We are given the opportunity to change so we don't create more destruction or repeat the same destruction in the future. Step Nine teaches us to use greater caution when choosing our actions.

The importance of being vigilant with practicing our program is fundamental in the Tenth Step. Through the use of a daily inventory, we can determine the best way to incorporate spiritual principles into our everyday actions. In the Tenth Step, we learn to immediately and sometimes proactively honor our values and spirits as we interact with others.

The consciousness and quiet reflection that is so basic to the Eleventh Step teaches us about the source of our spirits. In this step, we learn how to seek and honor the guidance we need in the care of our spirits.

After our spirits are awakened through the process of working and practicing the previous eleven steps, we embrace the Twelfth Step. It is with this essential step that we learn about our responsibility to make the message of recovery visible and available to anyone. We learn that spiritual principles are useless unless we practice them in our daily life.

Granted, these brief descriptions of some of the principles embodied in the steps do not begin to address the awesome power to effect change in our lives that each of them hold. The spirituality of character is the result of working, writing, and internalizing all the steps. Spirituality is the visible awakening found in the Twelfth Step. It gives us a positive view of ourselves, a strong sense of connection to the world, a sense of purpose in our lives, peace, and a healthy concern for ourselves and others. It usually means we can see how our concern for others results in benefits for us.

Spiritual awakenings that come as a result of working and internalizing the steps also help us to see ourselves as whole beings. This lets us think, feel, and act as who we are in spirit. It makes it easier for us to see that everything we think, feel, and do has an effect on our spirit and lets us use greater care with these parts of our lives.

Stewardship

The careful and responsible management
of something entrusted to one's care.

*Merriam-Webster's Collegiate Dictionary**

• • •

"WE DON'T OWN OUR TIME, IT'S GIVEN TO US
TO USE WISELY AS WE WALK ON THE EARTH.
MOST PEOPLE FIND IT EASY TO THINK OF TIME IN THIS WAY,
BUT IT'S HARDER TO THINK OF TALENTS AND TREASURES
AS THINGS WE DON'T OWN, AREN'T ENTITLED TO,
AND HAVE NO RIGHT TO HOARD.
STEWARDSHIP INVOLVES THOUGHTFUL CONSUMPTION
OF RESOURCES SO ALL WILL HAVE ENOUGH
AND THE PROCESSES THAT SUSTAIN LIFE WILL NOT BE HARMED."

THE REVEREND ROBERT BLEZARD, STEWARDSHIP OF LIFE INSTITUTE**

If we believe we are powerless over the disease of addiction and that we have gained freedom from this disease through a program of recovery, then it follows that everything we are and everything we have is something entrusted to our care.

Many of us, who have little trouble being good stewards of our belongings, find we struggle with being good stewards of our time and talents. Some of us have less trouble being good stewards of our time and talents, but find we have problems with stewardship of our belongings. Still others have difficulty seeing how they are responsible to steward anything they are or have since they firmly believe it is "mine" or "I worked for it."

We can, however, grow no matter where we find ourselves with stewardship. Accepting our needs and the benefits we get from the stewardship of others is often a good place to start. We ask ourselves, "What have I received in life that was good for me and completely unearned or undeserved?" If we are honest, the answer to this question begins with "my recovery" and is likely far longer than we would expect. We then ask ourselves, "How did this good thing I did not earn or deserve come to be in my life?" The answer to this question usually involves acknowledging the good stewardship of someone else.

Just as good stewardship has benefited us, we should do all we can to be good stewards and pass on the benefits.

MEDITATIVE THOUGHT

Help me see the richness in my life
in terms of its benefits to me
and the responsibility
I have as a steward.

Strong

Powerful and difficult to resist or defeat;
(of an argument or case) likely to succeed because
of sound reasoning or convincing evidence;
able to withstand force, pressure, or wear;
not easily affected by disease or hardship;
not easily disturbed, upset, or affected; very intense.

*Oxford Dictionary of English**

• • •

"BE AS A TOWER, THAT, FIRMLY SET;
SHAKES NOT ITS TOP FOR ANY BLAST THAT BLOWS."

DANTE ALIGHIERI

In active addiction, we may have been persistent, stubborn, or reckless, but we were not strong, in part, because we were powerless over our disease. We have the opportunity to be strong in recovery by working a program that gives us access to the power we need to live free of addiction. When we do this, we are able to acknowledge our inability to recover alone, but understand we can recover with the strength we gain from the principles of the program, meetings, our sponsor, and others. We know there is no permanent solution to our powerlessness, only a daily reprieve. We learn to use that reprieve to grow and change. We learn to rely on it, but we do not take it for granted.

Being strong gives us the ability to act on our assets even when we feel fear. We use our strength of character to examine and learn from things we have done. Strength sometimes requires performing difficult or new behavior or digging deep within ourselves to find the patience, commitment, and energy to do something right.

In strength of character, we are able to withstand force, pressure, and wear in our daily lives without surrendering to the easier, but less ideal solution. Being strong also means recognizing that sometimes the easiest solution is the best, and that being strong does not mean we should use our strength in every situation.

The gifts of strength are many. We become gentler with ourselves and others, we feel calmer, safer, and more capable. We are able to do things we first thought impossible and appreciate our strength. We learn we are far more competent than we imagined, and at the same time, we humbly recognize that none of what we are able to do would be possible without the gift of recovery. When we are able to see ourselves this way, we can take pride in what we do. We get to feel satisfied and good about ourselves without the unhealthy pride of ego.

MEDITATIVE THOUGHT

HELP ME BE STRONG ENOUGH
TO BE GENTLE WITH MYSELF AND OTHERS.
HELP ME USE MY STRENGTH
TO SELECT THE PERSONAL ASSET
MOST APPROPRIATE TO THE SITUATION.

Trusting

Showing or tending to have a belief in a person's
honesty or sincerity; not suspicious.

*Oxford Dictionary of English** *

• • •

"YOU NEED NOT WRESTLE FOR YOUR GOOD.
YOUR GOOD FLOWS TO YOU MOST EASILY
WHEN YOU ARE RELAXED, OPEN, AND TRUSTING."

ALAN COHEN**

In active addiction, being trusting rarely would have worked for us. The isolation, insanity, and stark interior landscape of addiction are not fertile ground for trust. Many of us come into recovery beaten, confused, angry, and alone. As we do the things required of us to recover, we begin to trust the people who help us, the program, and our higher power. This often provides us with the reassurance we need to trust the world.

The trust of character is the open-hearted faith that eventually all things work out for the best. Sometimes trust is a matter of giving someone the benefit of the doubt. Other times trust requires us to step into the unknown and try something outside our comfort zone.

The trust of character is not just what we do; it is the attitude

*By permission of Oxford University Press. © 1998, 1999, 2001, 2003 by Oxford University Press.
**From "Daily Inspirations" by Alan Cohen. Used by permission. All rights reserved.
For more information on Alan Cohen's books and programs, visit www.alancohen.com.

and intention with which we do it. If we give someone a chance, but then look for a way to control them, we are not trusting. If we jealously guard our personality and abilities to protect ourselves from being known or from unwanted attention, we are not trusting. If we take more than reasonable care for every action or choice we make, we are not trusting.

The benefits of being trusting are far-reaching. Being trusting lets us simplify our lives by showing up, doing the best we can, and then relaxing and enjoying whatever happens. Trust gives us the freedom to let others into our lives. Trust gives us the peace and comfort we need to enjoy relationships and the opportunities we have to help others. Trust keeps us in touch with our connections and our place in the world.

MEDITATIVE THOUGHT

As I live, help me trust.
Help me trust the process of recovery,
the people in my life, myself, and the world.
Help me notice and enjoy
the peace and calm that flow from trusting.

Trustworthy

Able to be relied on as honest or truthful.
*Oxford Dictionary of English**

• • •

"THE CHIEF LESSON I HAVE LEARNED
IN A LONG LIFE IS THAT THE ONLY WAY
YOU CAN MAKE A MAN TRUSTWORTHY
IS TO TRUST HIM; AND THE SUREST WAY
TO MAKE HIM UNTRUSTWORTHY
IS TO DISTRUST HIM."

HENRY L. STIMSON

Being trustworthy was seldom considered an asset for most of us in active addiction. Usually we most often could be trusted to do hurtful, wrong, or confusing things. We did these things for reasons not readily apparent to anyone, including ourselves. This behavior led most people with whom we were in contact to believe we were not trustworthy. We may have felt badly about their view of us. We even may have longed to be able to behave and be treated as trustworthy, but as using addicts, this was not possible.

Once we have freedom from active addiction, we often are told to "just do the next right thing." If we heed this suggestion enough, we become trustworthy over time. As we notice others rightfully placing trust in us, we begin to trust ourselves. As this happens we feel better about our lives and our choices. This is one of the most important foundations of character.

The trustworthiness of character is the ability to act consistent with our values without regard for the actions of others or external circumstances. When we are trustworthy, we do not seek to excuse or avoid our choices or their consequences by blaming or diverting attention to others. Being trustworthy makes us accountable for our actions. This is one of the greatest opportunities for growth and protection in recovery. If we are able to listen with an open mind to what we are being asked or told, we have the opportunity to grow or recognize potential reservations in our program before we relapse or cause pain and destruction in our lives.

The gifts of trustworthiness are many. They include a sense of peace and safety, the sense of genuine connection with others, and the satisfaction of days well lived and challenges well answered.

MEDITATIVE THOUGHT

HELP ME DO WHAT'S RIGHT CONSISTENTLY ENOUGH
TO BE TRUSTWORTHY. HELP ME BE WILLING
TO EXAMINE MY CHOICES AND ACTIONS AND TO KNOW MYSELF BETTER.
HELP ME NOTICE AND BE GRATEFUL FOR THE GIFTS
THAT FLOW FROM MY BEING TRUSTWORTHY.

Unpretentious

Not attempting to impress others
with an appearance of greater importance,
talent, or culture than is actually possessed.

Oxford Dictionary of English*

• • •

"LIKE FIRE, MONEY ITSELF IS NEITHER GOOD NOR EVIL.
IT IS NEUTRAL, ITS CHARACTER DETERMINED BY
THE EYE OF THE PERCEIVER, THE HAND OF THE USER."

JERROLD MUNDIS, *MAKING PEACE WITH MONEY***

While using, we often sought to impress others, keep them at a distance, or service our disease by trying to appear better or worse than we really were. When we see ourselves defined by our differences, we isolate ourselves. In recovery, we learn that even when we are different, we can choose to focus on what we have in common with others. When we focus on how we are like others, we make emotional connections to them that make it easier to ask for and offer help.

Over time, we begin to see our differences are only important in the opportunities they offer us to deepen our connections. We see that who we are, the ways we are different, and the ways we are the same have been given to us by our higher power. Even as we work for financial security, education, or good behavior, we often see our ability is something we were born with, not something we earned.

We can only take credit and feel satisfaction in the ways we have used what we have been given. When we consider this, being or acting pretentious is nearly impossible, and everything we are and have becomes an extension of the gifts given to us.

MEDITATIVE THOUGHT

HELP ME ASK THESE QUESTIONS SO THAT
I MAY REMAIN UNPRETENTIOUS:
"WHAT HAVE I DONE WITH THE ABILITIES I HAVE BEEN GIVEN?
IN WHAT WAYS HAVE I CONTRIBUTED TO MY OWN RECOVERY?
TO OTHERS? TO THE WORLD?"

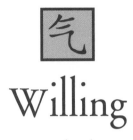

Willing

Eager or prepared to do something.
Oxford Dictionary of English*

• • •

"EVEN IF STRENGTH FAILS, BOLDNESS AT LEAST WILL DESERVE PRAISE:
IN GREAT ENDEAVORS EVEN TO HAVE HAD THE WILL IS ENOUGH."

SEXTUS PROPERTIUS

Most of us spent our active addiction feeling like victims of the whims of the world. Our lives were controlled by our disease and whatever willingness we had to grow or change was perverted. We may have done new and reckless things in order to get or use drugs, but we did not do them from a place of willingness, but as slaves to our disease.

In recovery, when we get freedom from our obsessive thoughts and compulsive actions, we become willing. First we become willing to do whatever it takes to stay clean, and then we develop a willingness to be honest and realistic about our lives in active addiction. When we look honestly at the mess we made of our lives before recovery, most of us are able to see a substantial change was needed.

Seeing the need for change helps us do the strange, new, and sometimes frightening things we are asked to do to stay clean. Some, however, whose lives have been more badly damaged and who need recovery as bad as or worse than we do, never develop the willingness to change. It appears that some part of the feeling or motivation of willingness is a gift and outside our control.

The sense that when we became willing we were given an unearned gift may bother us. We may feel insecure—that having been given it, we may also be at risk of losing it. We may be bothered by the unfairness of having received something others were denied. However, the only action we can take is to honor and nurture our willingness and try to share it with others.

Nurturing our willingness means working a program of recovery. It requires that we attend meetings, work with a sponsor, and write steps. Then, when we have experience, strength, and hope, we share it and look for ways to be of service in our recovery fellowship and the world. Acting in willingness requires that we do what we know to be right even when we don't feel like it.

This means we consider our thoughts and feelings as we become physically, intellectually, emotionally, and spiritually balanced in recovery. All of who we are should be considered in what we do with respect to willingness. If we are tired or afraid when we are called to help another addict, willingness helps us get out of bed.

Wisdom

The quality of having experience,
knowledge, and good judgment.

Oxford Dictionary of English*

• • •

"KNOWLEDGE, A RUDE UNPROFITABLE MASS,
THE MERE MATERIALS WITH WHICH WISDOM BUILDS,
TILL SMOOTHED AND SQUARED AND FITTED TO ITS PLACE,
DOES BUT ENCUMBER WHOM IT SEEMS TO ENRICH.
KNOWLEDGE IS PROUD THAT HE HAS LEARNED SO MUCH;
WISDOM IS HUMBLE THAT HE KNOWS NO MORE."

WILLIAM COWPER

In active addiction, we may have had experience and knowledge, but our judgment was almost always clouded by the fog of our disease. At times we may have been able to avoid disaster by using experience or knowledge or by following our instinct, but few of us were wise. The definition above makes it clear that to be wise we must have three things in the same place at the same time. We must have experience, knowledge, and good judgment. Having any one or two of these attributes does not allow us to be wise because the wise think, feel, and act differently than the foolish.

Wisdom can be understood as "a process of sensing, thinking, feeling, considering our wants and needs, exploring our options, and then choosing and taking action," according to Dr. Robert E. Hunter, clinical director of the Problem Gambling Center in Las Vegas, who has worked in the field of addiction for more than twenty-five years.

The wise, after taking action, usually take inventory of how this worked for them by repeating the process while considering the consequences of their actions.

In recovery, this often means reviewing our thoughts with another recovering addict. After this review and when we believe our thinking is clear and complete, the wise check internally about what they are feeling. When we are clear about what we want or need, we can move on to considering options.

Once we have decided on the best option, we take action. Checking with another recovering addict what we are sensing, thinking, feeling, wanting or needing, considering, or doing is often required throughout this process. Addicts commonly go from sensing, to thinking, to taking action without addressing what they feel, what they want and need, or what their options may be. In recovery, by working the Twelve Steps and learning to listen to others, we may become better at wisdom.

Wisdom comes with many gifts. When we are wise we are better able to understand ourselves and others; we are better able to select approaches to problems; and we are better prepared and able to handle the consequences of our choices because we already have considered them.

MEDITATIVE THOUGHT

HELP ME USE ALL OF THE ABILITIES I HAVE
TO MAKE WISE DECISIONS ABOUT MY LIFE.
HELP ME NOTICE AND BE GRATEFUL
FOR THE GIFTS IN MY LIFE THAT FLOW FROM WISDOM.